American College of Physicians

Home Care Guide

for
Cancer

For Family and Friends Giving Care at Home.

Also Available from the American College of Physicians

Clinical Practice Guidelines

Common Diagnostic Tests: Use and Interpretation—Second Edition

Common Screening Tests

Diagnostic Strategies for Common Medical Problems

Drug Prescribing in Renal Failure—Third Edition

Guide for Adult Immunization—Third Edition

Publications from the *British Medical Journal* are now distributed in North America by the American College of Physicians.

Publications catalogue and ordering information for American College of Physicians and *British Medical Journal* publications are available from:

Customer Service

American College of Physicians

Independence Mall West

Sixth Street at Race

Philadelphia, PA 19106-1572

(215) 351-2600

(800) 523-1546

American College of Physicians

Home Care Guide

for
Cancer

For Family and Friends Giving Care at Home.

Editor
Peter S. Houts, PhD

Associate Editors
Arthur M. Nezu, PhD
Christine M. Nezu, PhD
Julia A. Bucher, RN, PhD, OCN
Allan Lipton, MD

Contributors
Dale B. Schelzel, RN, OCN
Sandra J. Spoljaric, RN, OCN
Kathy B. Kambic, RN, OCN
Elise M. Givant, RN, OCN
Georgia L. Trostle, RN, OCN
Glenda M. Trumpower, MSW
Carol D. Nolt, MSW
Eric J. Pfeiffer, BA

Project Coordinator
Carole A. Bean

Library of Congress Cataloging-in-Publication Data

American College of Physicians home care guide for cancer :
for family and friends giving care at home / Peter S. Houts, editor.
p. cm. – (American College of Physicians homecare guides)

Includes index.
ISBN 0-943126-30-4

1. Cancer–Patients–Home care. I. Houts, Peter S. II. American
College of Physicians. III. Title: Home care guide for cancer.
IV. Series.

[DNLM: 1. Home Nursing–methods–handbooks. 2. Neoplasms–nursing–handbooks.
WY 39 A5115 1994]
RC266.A62 1994
362.1'96994–dc20
DNLM/DLC
for Library of Congress

94-5995
CIP

Author proceeds from the sale of this book will be used to support research and educa-
tion to improve the quality of life of persons with cancer and family and friends involved
in their care.

Acknowledgments

Many persons have contributed to the development of the cancer home care plans. They include physicians, nurses, psychologists, and social workers, as well as persons with cancer and their family and friends. Several people have been especially generous in contributing their time and expertise and, as a result, have had a substantial influence on the development and growth of this project. We are deeply indebted to Regena Tripp, RN, OCN; David Houts; Charles Schreiber; Harold Harvey, MD; Bruce Nicholson, MD; and George Simms, MD.

The plans were reviewed and edited by cancer care professionals as well as by consumers. Their comments and editing have been invaluable. These include Bonnie Koch, RN, OCN; Carol Ann Peters, RN, MSN; Bruce Nicholson, MD; Diane Erdos, RN, MSN; Sharon Olson, RN, MSN; Irena Rusenas, MS; Eric Pfeiffer, BA; Margaret Davitt, RN, MSN; Susan A. Rokita, RN, MSN; Sandra Frey, RN, OCN; Shirley Faddis, MSN, OCN; Katherine Yoder, RN, OCN; Joan Hermann, ACSW; Diane Blum, ACSW; Carolyn Messner, ACSW; Mary Lander, RN; Barbara Robinawitz, PhD; Harold Piety; William Sattazahn, Jr.; Marion Sattazahn; Kenneth Kohler; Timothy Freer; Edward Henry; Marjorie Cassel; and Marion Spangler. We appreciate the help of Barbara Van Horn and Renee Atchison Ziegler of the Institute for the Study of Adult Literacy in editing the manuscript to maximize readability of the home care plans and the help of Pat Wieland for the layout and design of this book.

We also want to express our appreciation to the following people for their support and suggestions during this project: Harold Harvey, MD; John Stryker, MD; Frank Davidoff, MD, FACP; Thomas Feagin, MD, FACP; Charles Lewis, MD, FACP; Arthur Ulene, MD; Nick Leasure, MD; David Hufford, PhD; Steven Hulse, MEd; Judy Lyter, RN, BS; Nancy Toth, RN, BSN; Catherine Kleese, RN, OCN; Mary Jo Templin, RN; Janice Mills, RN, MS; Bonnie Bixler, MEd; and Julia Yost.

Administrative support from our host institutions has been invaluable in carrying out this work and is greatly appreciated. These include the Department of Behavioral Science and the Oncology Division of the Department of Medicine of the Pennsylvania State University College of Medicine; the Division of Clinical Psychology of the Department of Mental Health Sciences of Hahnemann University; and the Department of Nursing of Bloomsburg University.

While each home care plan was reviewed and edited by many persons, certain people played special roles by contributing significantly to the first versions of the plans and by actively participating in their revisions and final editing. They are:

Dale Schelzel RN, OCN: *Nausea and Vomiting, Tiredness and Fatigue, Problems with Veins, Fever and Infections, Problems with Bleeding, Problems with Appetite*;

Sandra Spoljaric, RN, OCN: *Problems with the Mouth, Hair Loss*;

Kathy Kambic, RN, OCN: *Diarrhea, Constipation*;

Elise Givant, RN, OCN; and Peter Houts, PhD: *Problems with Getting Information from Medical Staff*;

Georgia Trostle, RN, BSN; Bruce Nicholson, MD; and Julia Bucher, RN, PhD, OCN: *Cancer Pain*;

Carole Bean and Peter Houts, PhD: *Maintaining Positive Experiences*;

Sandra J. Spoljaric, RN, OCN; and Mary Lander, RN: *Skin Problems*;

Carol Nolt, MSW, and Julia Bucher, RN, PhD, OCN: *Getting Help from Community Agencies and Volunteer Groups*;

Eric Pfeiffer, MS; Arthur Nezu, PhD; Christine Nezu, PhD; and Peter Houts, PhD: *Coping with Anxiety, Coping with Depression*;

Julia Bucher, RN, PhD, OCN: *Coordinating Care from One Treatment Setting to Another, Moving around the House, Sexual Problems;* and

Peter Houts, PhD: *Getting Companionship and Support from Family and Friends.*

The "Succeeding at Caregiving" home care plan was adapted by Peter S. Houts, PhD; Carol Nolt, MSW; Glenda Trumpower, MSW; and Julia Bucher, RN, PhD, for cancer caregivers from the "Caring Families" manual developed by the Family Caregiver Project at the University of North Carolina at Charlotte. The authors of the "Caring Families" manual were D.D. Fernald, PhD; James R. Cook, PhD; and Catherine A. Gutman, DrPH, RN. Its development was supported by grant no. 90PD0153 from the Office of Human Development Services of the U.S. Department of Health and Human Services.

Other important sources of information included *Helping People Cope: A Guide for Families Facing Cancer* developed by the Cancer Control Program of the Pennsylvania Department of Health and authored by Joan F. Hermann, ACSW; Sandra L. Wojtkowiak, RN, BSN; Peter S. Houts, PhD; and S. Benham Kahn, MD, as well as many informational booklets and brochures developed and distributed by the National Cancer Institute and the American Cancer Society.

The Cancer Home Care Plans Project

The Cancer Home Care Plans project was initiated by a bequest from Elizabeth G. Holmes to the Pennsylvania State University College of Medicine. After her death from cancer, Mrs. Holmes' family requested that the funds be used to help families of persons with cancer. Peter S. Houts, PhD, was appointed project director. The first project activity was a literature review on how cancer affects families. This review showed that one of the principal needs of family and friends caring for a person with cancer was for more information and guidance for dealing with the physical, psychological, and social problems that result from the illness. To address this need, Dr. Houts collaborated with Dr. Arthur Nezu and Dr. Christine Nezu of Hahnemann University and Dr. Julia Bucher of Bloomsburg University in designing home care plans to guide home caregivers through a series of problem-solving steps in dealing with common physical, emotional, and social problems, which people with cancer and caregivers may experience during the illness. Over fifty cancer care professionals, persons with cancer, and family members and friends involved in their care collaborated in writing twenty-two home care plans. The plans were extensively field tested in several different oncology treatment settings and with a wide variety of users. Their suggestions and comments were incorporated into the final plans. Additional support during the development and field testing stages was provided by the Central Pennsylvania Oncology Group, Schering Corporation, the Cancer Control Program of the Pennsylvania Department of Health, and grant 1 R25 CA57938 from the National Cancer Institute.

Table of Contents

Solving Problems Using the Home Care Guide for Cancer

Now, more than ever, we are winning the fight against cancer. Scientific and technical advances in cancer medicine have increased the chances of extending life and have even increased the chance of cure for most types of cancer. Furthermore, there have been important advances in controlling symptoms and side effects of treatment so that the quality of life of people with cancer can be better now than it ever was in the past.

But these advances in cancer treatment have also made cancer care more complex. Treatment often includes surgery, radiation therapy, and chemotherapy. Frequent tests are often required to monitor the effects of treatment. And cancer treatments often go on for months and then must be resumed if the disease comes back. As a result, persons with cancer and their families must be prepared to cope with a wide range of physical, emotional, and social consequences of the disease and treatments for extended periods of time. In addition, as time in the hospital is shortened and as more and more treatments are given in the doctor's office or clinic, family caregivers are taking on more responsibility for providing care. Therefore, family caregivers have become important members of the health care team. They are assuming many caregiving responsibilities that, until recently, had been carried out by health professionals. Health professionals now rely on family caregivers, not only to provide support and encouragement to the person with cancer, but also to manage medications, help control symptoms and side effects, and report problems that require professional intervention.

It is our experience that home caregivers can carry out these responsibilities very well, if they have clear guidance from health professionals. Since family caregivers are members of the health care team, they need to deal with problems the same way that other team members do and to work cooperatively with health professionals. The home care plans give this guidance. They have been written by cancer care professionals with many years of experience and with help from home caregivers and persons with cancer. The plans give you the information you need to solve problems, including understanding the problem, when to get professional help, what you can do on your own, possible obstacles, and how to carry out and adjust the plan. This is the same kind of information that health professionals use to solve medical problems.

The home care plans also help health professionals to monitor and guide care that is given at home. If family caregivers follow these plans, then professional staff know that family caregivers are following procedures recommended by cancer care professionals. Furthermore, since the plans tell when to call for professional help, staff can be assured that, if the plans are followed, they will be kept informed when problems need their attention.

But this program isn't just for caregivers. People with cancer should also read the home care guide book. They need to understand the plans and to participate in carrying them out if they are to be successful. Furthermore, people with cancer are often their own caregivers—for example, when they are living alone or when family and friends rely on them for directions. If you are a person with cancer, we suggest that, when you read this workbook, you think of yourself as your own caregiver.

There are four key ideas that will help you to be effective in solving your caregiving problems and to make the best use of the home care guide book.

You can remember these four key ideas by thinking of the word COPE:

C **for Creativity**

O **for Optimism**

P **for Planning**

E **for Expert information**

The following pages discuss these four ideas in detail.

Get EXPERT INFORMATION about the Problem and What You Can Do about It

The foundation for good problem solving is knowledge about the problem and about what can be done to deal with the problem. The home care plans give you five kinds of expert information needed to solve caregiving problems.

Understanding the problem

Define the problem, who is most likely to have it, what can be done to help, and what you can reasonably hope to achieve.

When to get professional help

When to call health care professionals, including when you should call immediately and when you can wait until regular office hours.

What you can do to help

What you can do on your own to deal with the problem and what you can do to prevent the problem from happening or becoming severe.

Possible obstacles

Common attitudes and misinformation that can interfere with carrying out the home care plan as well as how to deal with these obstacles.

Carrying out and adjusting your plan

How to check on whether the plan is working and what to do if it isn't.

Read the home care plans *before* starting to deal with a problem—then you will have a complete understanding of the problem and what you can do to deal with it. You should also re-read the plan periodically, especially if your plan does not seem to be working, to be sure that you are doing everything you can.

Develop an Orderly and Systematic PLAN

Problem solving is done best in an orderly, systematic way. This means you should:

Get the facts

Be clear about what is happening. Separate facts from opinions.

Review what you can do

Read the home care plan and other written information about the problem. Ask health professionals for recommendations. Think back over your own experiences for ideas and strategies that worked in the past. Ask what you can reasonably hope to achieve.

Decide on the best strategy

Compare the advantages and disadvantages of the different approaches you could take, and develop a strategy that has a reasonable chance of achieving your goal.

Consider obstacles

Think of what could interfere with your plan, and think creatively about what you can do to deal with those obstacles.

Carry out and adjust your plan

Set deadlines for yourself to be sure things get done. Keep records of how the plan is working. This will help you to monitor progress and to explain to medical staff what you have done and what the results were. If the plan is not working or you are not having as much success as you hoped, ask yourself if you are expecting change too fast and whether you should adjust your goals. Then repeat the problem-solving steps to develop a new plan, paying special attention to maintaining a positive attitude and expecting success.

Have an OPTIMISTIC Attitude while Being Realistic about Your Problems

Have a positive attitude

<u>One of the most important things you can do to help the person you are caring for is to have a positive attitude.</u> People who are dealing with the stress of cancer and cancer treatments need encouragement, and they need help noticing the good things that are happening. The home care plan for Maintaining Positive Experiences has suggestions for how to do this. At the same time, it is important to be realistic about the seriousness of their problems so that they do not feel that their problems are being ignored or belittled.

Expect to succeed

If you think that there is a good chance of succeeding, you will do your best. If you think the problem is hopeless and that nothing will work, it will be hard for you to do your best at carrying out your plans, and the people who are around you will become discouraged, too. If you do feel discouraged and negative, then get help from someone who has a positive attitude and who is a good problem solver. This could be the person with cancer, friends or family members, or health professionals. Read the home care plan for Coping with Depression for help in controlling negative thinking that interferes with effective problem solving.

Take breaks from caregiving

<u>Do things that you enjoy so that you will be able to have a positive outlook, even when you feel under stress.</u> Read the home care plan for Succeeding at Caregiving for ideas and guidance about how to deal with your feelings as a caregiver. Also, the home care plans for Maintaining Positive Experiences, Getting Companionship and Support from Family and Friends, Coping with Anxiety, and Coping with Depression apply as much to you as they do to the person with

cancer. Read and use those plans for yourself. They will help you to have the emotional strength you need to have a positive attitude and to solve the problems that come with caregiving.

Be CREATIVE

As a caregiver you will be constantly challenged to think creatively

Each person is unique and each problem is unique. Therefore, you must be creative in adapting your plans to fit each unique situation.

Most plans will run into obstacles or road blocks. Overcoming or side-stepping these obstacles will also challenge your creativity. <u>When your plans don't work out as you had hoped, you should see this as a challenge to your creativity</u>.

Here are three things you can do to help yourself think creatively when dealing with obstacles:

1. <u>See the obstacle from someone else's point of view</u>. Put yourself in the shoes of another person who can look at your problem differently and ask yourself what he or she would do.

2. <u>Ask other people</u> who have faced similar problems for ideas about how to get around your obstacle.

3. <u>Ask how important or serious the obstacle really is</u>. Does this obstacle really stop you from carrying out your plan? Sometimes you can ignore or work around an obstacle and still carry out your plan.

How To Develop Your Own Home Care Plans

The home care plans in this manual deal with only the most common problems that people with cancer and their home caregivers have. You can also use the same home care plans as models for the information you need to solve other caregiving problems.

Understanding the problem

The first step in developing your own home care plan is to understand exactly what the problem is you are trying to solve. You should also have a clear idea of your goal.

You need to find out what kinds of people have this problem, when they have it, what kinds of things can be done to help, and what is a reasonable goal to work toward. For medical problems, ask the doctor or nurse. For nonmedical problems, social workers and nurses are often very knowledgeable. Other caregivers and members of support groups can also help.

You also need to know the facts for your situation. Exactly what happened, when did it happen, how often did it happen, how severe is it, what was done in the past, and what were the results? Be sure that these are facts and not just opinions or impressions. Facts are the foundation for successful problem solving.

When to get professional help

For medical problems or problems that could endanger the health of the person with cancer, ask the doctor, nurse, or social worker when and whom you should call.

What you can do to help

For medical problems, ask the doctor, nurse, or social worker what you can do on your own to deal with the problem—or to prevent it from happening.

For nonmedical problems, you can develop your own strategies by using your experience and your creativity and by asking other people for ideas. Think back to what you did in the past that was helpful for similar problems. If something was just partly successful, think how you could use it with this problem. Be creative. Try to think of new ways to look at the problem and unusual ways to solve it. Try "brainstorming," where you free your imagination and try to think of unusual ideas. When you brainstorm, make the longest list of ideas you can, and don't criticize your ideas until after the list is finished. Then choose the best ideas from the list. The freer your imagination and the longer the list, the better are your chances of coming up with a creative solution. Finally, you should weigh the advantages and disadvantages of each idea and choose what to do based on your past experiences and what you think will have the best chance of succeeding.

Possible obstacles

Consider what could prevent you from carrying out your plan and how you are going to deal with these obstacles.

For medical problems, ask the doctor, nurse, or social worker about difficulties that other people have had in dealing with the problem and how to overcome them.

For nonmedical problems, think of what obstacles could prevent you from carrying out your plan and how you will deal with them.

Carrying out and adjusting your plan

And, finally, you need to know how to monitor your progress. What changes should you be looking for and how fast should you realistically expect to see change? Ask health professionals or people who have dealt with similar problems for suggestions and advice.

How To Make the Best Use of Home Care Plans

First read the outline headings to know what information the plan contains. Then read the whole plan to fully understand what you can do and why.

The first page of each plan is an overview of what is in the home care plan. This gives you a road map of what is in the plan. The home care plans are organized as outlines. You can quickly read the topic headings in bold type and have a good overview of what the plans are saying. Topics with an arrow in front of them are actions you can take or symptoms you can look for. So, if you want to quickly review what you can do, just read the topics with arrows to the left.

We also recommend that you read all the information in a home care plan before you start dealing with a problem. Then you will have a complete understanding of the problem and what you can do to solve it.

Notice and deal with problems early

One of the most important ways that you can help the person with cancer is to notice and deal with problems early. Problems are easier to solve when they are just starting, and early intervention can often prevent problems from becoming serious. If you read the home care plans *before* problems develop, you will be prepared if they occur, and, since some plans include how to prevent problems, you can even prevent some problems from happening.

Succeeding at Caregiving

Overview of the
Home Care Plan for Succeeding at Caregiving

Understanding the Problem

Successful caregivers are problem solvers

They work with other people to solve problems

They have a positive attitude toward caregiving

They take care of themselves

When To Get Professional Help

If you are experiencing severe anxiety or depression

If communication between you and the person with cancer has broken down

If your relationship with the person with cancer is clouded by a history of abuse or addiction

What You Can Do To Be a Successful Caregiver

Work and communicate effectively with the person with cancer

Take care of your own needs and feelings

Possible Obstacles

"He doesn't want to talk about feelings."

"What if she talks about things that I don't want to hear?"

"She won't follow my advice."

"I don't have time to take care of my needs."

"If I don't do it, it won't get done."

"I hate to ask other people to help me."

"The person I'm helping doesn't want anyone else to help."

Carrying Out and Adjusting Your Plan

Start now—use these strategies early to have strength and support when you need it

Be realistic in your expectations for sharing feelings

Be realistic about what you expect of yourself

Ask for help before you feel overwhelmed

(Topics with an arrow in front of them are actions you can take or symptoms you can look for.)

Succeeding at Caregiving

Understanding the Problem

Successful caregivers are successful problem solvers

Caregiving involves solving problems. You have been solving problems throughout your life. The only difference now is that many of the problems that come with cancer are new to you and to the person you are helping. The home care plans will help both of you to solve these new problems; they will give you information and guidance organized in the steps you need to take to solve the problem.

The plans are designed to help you solve problems, but you and the person with cancer are the ones who will actually solve the problems. You decide what actions to take. You adjust the plans to meet your special situations. You carry out the plans. And you monitor how well the plans are working and make changes as needed. You also must develop new plans on your own to deal with problems that are not in this workbook.

You and the person you are helping are in charge of dealing with your problems. You are not people who are just following instructions but are people who are making decisions and taking actions.

Successful caregivers work with other people to solve problems

The successful caregiver is also a team player—working with the person with cancer, working with other family and friends, and working with medical staff to solve problems.

The person with cancer is central to the team. Success in carrying out home care plans requires his or her participation and agreement. Furthermore, the person with cancer has a right to participate in his or her own care and should be involved in all problem-solving discussions that affect him or her.

Health care professionals are also key members of the team. Caregivers work with them to ensure that the care given at home is consistent with the best medical practices. Since health professionals played a key role in developing the home care plans, you can be sure that, if you are following these plans, you are giving the best possible care. Health professionals are also a valuable source of information and advice about how to handle nonmedical problems that come with the illness.

Family members and friends who share in caregiving are also important team members. In addition to helping in practical ways, they give encouragement and emotional support, and they can share their experiences with and knowledge of dealing with similar problems in their lives.

Successful caregivers have a positive attitude toward caregiving

Successful caregivers emphasize the positive parts of caregiving. For example, some successful caregivers see their work as helping someone they love and care deeply about. Others see caregiving spiritually—"I think this is part of God's plan for me." Others feel that caregiving has enriched their lives. Others see it as a challenge and want to do the best job they can. And some see caregiving as a way of showing appreciation for the love and care they have received themselves.

Caregiving can have important benefits. Caring for someone can give you a sense of satisfaction and confidence. Families who do caregiving often feel closer to each other and to the person who is ill. You can also find new, rewarding friendships with other caregivers who are going through similar experiences. And you may discover inner strengths that you didn't realize you had.

You can also use the illness to open doors to new friends and relationships. This can happen from talking to other people who have faced the same problems, from meeting people at a support group, from meeting people who have volunteered to help with caregiving, and from family members and old friends who have grown distant but who are drawn together because of the illness.

Successful caregivers take care of themselves

Helping someone who is going through cancer treatments can be difficult and stressful. The more you take care of your own need for rest, food, enjoyment, and relaxation, the better you will be able to help the person with cancer. The home care plans for Maintaining Positive Experiences and Getting Companionship and Support from Family and Friends apply as much to you as to the person you are helping. Use the ideas in those plans for yourself to be able to do your best as a caregiver.

Your goals for being a successful caregiver are:

1. To be an effective team player working with the person with cancer, health professionals, and family members and friends in solving home care problems, and

2. To take care of your own needs during this illness so that you have the emotional strength to be an effective caregiver.

When To Get Professional Help

Ask for help from a doctor, nurse, social worker, member of the clergy, or other professional if any of the following conditions exist:

➤ **You are experiencing severe anxiety or depression.** Read the home care plans for Coping with Anxiety and Coping with Depression for a list of anxiety and depression symptoms, which indicate that professional help is needed.

➤ **Communication between you and the person with cancer has broken down or has become painful or difficult.** The stresses that come with cancer physical, psychological, financial, and emotional—can hamper your ability to communicate with the person you are caring for. If anxiety and stress levels have risen to where you aren't able to talk openly with the person with cancer about important issues, you should get professional help from a counselor, member of the clergy, hospital social worker, or hospice staff member.

➤ **Your relationship with the person with cancer is clouded by a history of abuse or addiction.** Caregivers who have suffered through verbal, mental, physical, or sexual abuse from the persons they are caring for, or where alcohol or drug addiction has affected relationships, are likely to have serious problems in caregiving. They already have strong and deep-seated feelings, usually built up over many years. This situation calls for professional help from the start.

What You Can Do To Be a Successful Caregiver

Working and communicating effectively with the person with cancer

This is your most important job. It can also be the most challenging. The person you are caring for has to deal with the physical effects of the disease and treatments as well as with the psychological and social challenges of living with cancer. This may make it difficult for him or her to participate in the home care plans. Nonetheless, <u>your job is to involve the person you are caring for as much as possible in making decisions and carrying out the plans.</u>

➤ **Help the person with cancer to deal with the diagnosis emotionally and to live as normal a life as possible.** Some people with cancer try to deal with upsetting news by pretending that it didn't happen. This can be healthy when it helps them live as normal a life as possible. It can be harmful, however, if they do things that make the illness worse, such as avoiding treatment or doing activities that are physically harmful.

Support the efforts of the person with cancer to live as normal a life as possible. But, if he or she is pretending that nothing is wrong, you need to be clear in your own mind about what is really happening. This is when your objectivity is important to be sure that he or she is benefiting from pretending and does not do things that could be harmful.

➤ **Create a climate that encourages sharing feelings and that supports his or her efforts to share.** Talk about important or sensitive topics in a time and place that's calm and conducive to open communication—not in the midst of a crisis or a family argument. If your time for talking in your family is around the dinner table, that's the time to do it now. Try to think: When have you had important talks in the past? Strive to recreate that setting.

Communicate your availability. One of the most important messages you can communicate to the person with cancer is this: "If you want to discuss this uncomfortable issue, I'm willing to do it." But leave the timing up to the person with cancer. To the greatest extent possible, let decisions on what feelings to share and when, how, and with whom to share them be up to the person with cancer. By not pressing the issue, you allow the person to retain control over part of his or her life at a time when many issues and decisions are beyond his or her control.

➤ **Understand that men and women often communicate in different ways, and make allowances for those differences.** Although there are many exceptions, women often express their feelings more openly than men in our society. If you're a male caregiver and the person with cancer is a woman, be aware that, when she shares feelings, you may find yourself giving advice when she wants support and understanding. If you're a female caregiver and the person with cancer is male, be aware that he may express his feelings differently than you would. Pay special attention when he talks about things that are important to him.

> **Be realistic and flexible about what you hope to communicate or agree on.** People with cancer want to share many things, but they may not share them all with just one person. Let the person talk about whatever he or she wants with whomever he or she wants. It's OK if the person isn't telling you everything, as long as he or she is telling somebody. Also, remember that a person may have spent a lifetime developing a communications style, and that won't change overnight.

Sharing doesn't always mean talking. The person with cancer may feel more comfortable writing about his or her feelings or expressing them through an activity. He or she may express feelings in other nonverbal ways, such as by making gestures or expressions, touching, or just asking that you be present.

Remember that you don't have to agree. Two people aren't always at the same place at the same time. You and the person with cancer may disagree on issues such as when, how, and what to share, but remember that this is one of the patterns of life that can't always be resolved. If the person with cancer is your spouse, think back to times when one partner was ready to take a step—like starting a family—but the other was not. There's no simple answer to this; just be aware of it, and don't knock yourself out if you can't resolve every point.

When you and the person with cancer disagree on important issues

> **Explain your needs openly.** Sometimes you may need to ask him or her to do something to make your life easier or your caregiving responsibilities more manageable. Understand that conflict resolution doesn't always mean everybody's happy. On some issues, you'll have to give in, and on others, you'll have to ask him or her to give in.

> **Suggest a trial run or time limit.** If you want the person with cancer to try something (such as a new bed or a certain medication schedule) and he or she is resisting, ask to try it for a limited time, like a week, and then evaluate the situation. This avoids making the person feel locked into a decision. If the person resists writing a will or power of attorney, ask if he or she will at least read it over and discuss it.

> **Choose your battles carefully.** Ask yourself: "What's really important here? Am I being stubborn on an issue because I need to win an argument?" You can save energy by skipping the minor conflicts and using your energy and influence on issues that really count.

➤ **Let the person with cancer make decisions as much as possible.** A good example is when adult children living some distance away from a person with cancer want to move him or her into a nursing home. Although moving the person with cancer to a nursing home may make the adult child feel better, this may not be what the person with cancer wants. If the person with cancer understands the consequences (for example, no one may be around to help if he or she falls), the caregiver should accept the person's right to make that decision. Taking away a person's ability to make decisions can undermine feelings of control, which interferes with the ability to deal with other aspects of this stressful illness.

Taking care of your own needs and feelings

You need to be at your best if you are to do the best job of helping. Therefore, <u>you should pay attention to your own needs as well as those of the person you are helping</u>. Set limits on what you can reasonably expect yourself to do. You should take time off to care for yourself and your needs. And you should ask for help before stress builds up.

It is natural to have strong feelings when helping someone with a serious illness. Following is a list of common feelings that caregivers can have and strategies for dealing with them if they become severe.

Shock

<u>Caregivers as well as the person with cancer can feel overwhelmed and confused</u> when they first learn about the diagnosis of cancer or when they learn that the disease is not responding to treatment or is progressing. <u>Here are some things that other caregivers have done when they felt shocked and overwhelmed</u>:

➤ **Try not to make important decisions while you are upset.** Sometimes you must make decisions immediately, but often you don't have to. Ask the doctor, nurse, or social worker how long before a decision should be made.

➤ **Take time to sort things out.**

➤ **Talk over important problems** with others who are feeling more level-headed and rational. If you are feeling very upset or discouraged, then ask a friend, neighbor, or family member to help. They can bring a calmer perspective to the situation as well as new ideas and help in dealing with the problems you are facing.

Anger

There are plenty of reasons for you to become angry while you are caring for an ill person. For example, the person you are caring for may, at times, be demanding or irritating. Friends, family members, or professionals may not be as helpful or understanding as you would like. Some people feel angry because they feel that their religion has let them down. It is natural to be angry when your life has been turned upside down, which often happens with a serious illness like cancer.

These feelings are normal! It is all right to feel this way at times. It is what you do with your feelings that is important. The best way to deal with angry feelings is to recognize them, accept them, and find some way to express them appropriately. If you don't deal with your anger, it can get in the way of almost everything you do.

Here are some things that other caregivers have done to deal with their anger:

➤ **Try to see the situation from the other person's point of view** and understand why he or she acted that way. Recognize that other people are under stress, too, and that some people are better than others in dealing with stressful situations.

➤ **Express your anger in an appropriate way before it gets too severe.** If you wait until your anger is severe, it will impair your judgment, and you are likely to make other people angry in return.

➤ **Get away from the situation for awhile,** and try to cool off before you go back and deal with what made you angry.

➤ **Find safe ways to express your anger.** This can include such things as beating on a pillow, yelling out loud in a car or in a closed room, or doing some hard exercise. Sometimes it helps to vent anger with someone who is "safe"—who won't be offended or strike back.

➤ **Talk to someone about why you feel angry.** Explaining to another person why you feel angry often helps you to understand why you reacted as you did and to see your reactions in perspective.

Fear

You may become afraid when someone you care for deeply has a serious illness. You do not know what is in store for him or her or for yourself, and you may be fearful that you won't be able to handle what happens.

Here are some things that other caregivers have done to deal with their fears:

➤ **Learn as much as possible about what is happening and what may happen in the future.** This can reduce fear of the unknown and help you to be realistic so that you can prepare for the future. Talk with health professionals and with other people who have cared for someone with cancer to see if you are exaggerating the risks.

➤ **Read the home care plan for Coping with Anxiety.** The ideas and techniques in that plan can be used by you as well as by the person with cancer.

➤ **Talk to someone about your fears.** It often helps to explain why you feel fearful to an understanding person. This helps you to think through the reasons for your feelings. Also, talking to an understanding person will show you that other people understand and appreciate how you feel.

Loss and sorrow

A serious, life-threatening illness can bring on a great sense of loss and sorrow. You may feel sad that plans that you had for the future may not be fulfilled. You may feel the loss of the "normal" person and the "normal" things you did before this illness. Memories of how he or she used to be may make you sad. Here are some things that other caregivers have done to deal with these feelings:

➤ **Talk about your feelings of loss with other people who have had similar experiences.** People who have been caregivers for persons with serious illnesses will usually understand how you feel. Support groups are one way to find people who have had similar experiences and who can understand and appreciate your feelings.

➤ **Read the home care plan for Coping with Depression.** Feelings of loss are often part of feeling depressed. The ideas and techniques in this home care plan can be used by you as well as by the person you are caring for to help manage or prevent depression.

Guilt

Many people who care for someone with cancer feel guilty at some time during the illness. They may feel guilty because they think they did something to cause the cancer or because they should have recognized the cancer sooner. They may feel guilty for not doing a better job of caring for the person with cancer. They may feel guilty because they feel angry or upset with him or her. And they may feel guilty because they are well and the person they care deeply about is sick. Some people feel guilt almost out of habit. They have learned from childhood to feel guilty when something goes wrong.

Although feeling guilty is understandable, it can interfere with doing the best possible job of caregiving. Guilt makes you think only about what *you* did wrong, although most problems have many causes and what you did is only part of the reason for the problem. To solve a problem, you have to look objectively at *all* of the causes and then develop plans to deal with the whole problem. For example, if you feel anger toward the person you are caring for, this is partly because of what he or she did as well as what you did. To deal with the cause of the anger, you have to talk openly with him or her about what you *both* did—and not just feel guilty about what you did and about feeling angry.

Here are some things that other caregivers have done to deal with feelings of guilt:

➤ **Talk to people who have had similar experiences about what happened and how they felt.** It is often easier to see a situation objectively when it happens to someone else. This can give you a perspective on your own problems.

➤ **Don't expect yourself to be perfect.** Remember that you are human and will make mistakes from time to time.

➤ **Don't dwell on mistakes.** Accept mistakes and get beyond them as best you can. The home care plan for Coping with Depression has useful ideas for controlling repetitive, negative thoughts, such as guilt, and for pushing them aside with positive, constructive thoughts.

Remember: You are at your best to help the person with cancer when you feel your best. If feeling guilty makes you upset, it can interfere with being the best possible caregiver.

Possible Obstacles

Think about what could prevent you from carrying out your plan for being a successful caregiver.

Here are some things that have stood in the way of others' being successful caregivers

1. "He doesn't want to talk about feelings."

   Response: He is the best judge of that. Your job is to make sure the opportunities are there to share when he or she decides it is right.

2. "What if she talks about things that I don't want to hear?"

   Response: Even if what you hear hurts you, consider it in the larger picture of what it means to the person to be able to express it. Remember that you don't have to solve anything. You're helpful if you just listen.

3. "He won't follow my advice."

   Response: If you're feeling frustrated because the person with cancer won't follow your advice, try to understand how important it is for him or her to retain some control. You may know what's best for the person you are caring for, but realize that your job is support. Your job is not to make the decision for the person. If you have a dominant personality or have been the one to make decisions in your family, be prepared to practice letting go.

4. "I'm swamped with problems, so I don't have time to take care of my needs."

   Response: This is the most common reason that caregivers become exhausted. They become preoccupied with problems and don't pay attention to themselves. <u>You will be a better caregiver in the long run if you take the time, especially when stress is high, to do things that you enjoy and that relax you</u>.

5. "If I don't do it, it won't get done."

   Response: Yes, it will. No one is indispensable. <u>You should also sort out things that really need to be done versus what you would like to see done</u>. It's OK to let some things, like housework, slide a bit when you take on new responsibilities.

6. "I hate to ask other people to help me."

> Response: There are two ways around this problem. You can get together socially with people who could help and let them volunteer or you could have someone else ask for help for you. <u>Read the home care plan for Getting Companionship and Support from Family and Friends for ideas about how to make others' visits pleasant and rewarding</u>. Then they will want to visit and help.

7. "The person I'm helping doesn't want other people to help us."

> Response: Suggest trying to get help for just a short time, and then you both can talk over how it worked. Also, <u>explain that *you* need help, not him or her</u>.

Think of *other* obstacles that could interfere with carrying out your plan

What additional road blocks could get in the way of your being a successful caregiver? For example, will the person with cancer cooperate? Will other people help? How will you explain your needs to other people? Do you have the time and energy to carry out these responsibilities?

You need to develop plans for getting around these road blocks. Use the four COPE ideas (creativity, optimism, planning, and expert information) in developing your plans. See the chapter on Solving Home Care Problems at the beginning of the book for a discussion of how to use the four COPE ideas in overcoming your obstacles.

Carrying Out and Adjusting Your Plan

How will you carry out your plan?

Start using the ideas in this home care plan now. <u>Don't wait until you feel overwhelmed</u>. It is easier to develop good caregiving habits and attitudes early before problems get out of hand.

It is especially important to begin work early on the home care plans for Maintaining Positive Experiences and Getting Companionship and Support from Family and Friends. They apply to you, the caregiver, as much as to the person with cancer. These plans can give you the strength and resources to deal with stressful situations. Use them early, and then have the strength and support available when you need it.

Be realistic in your expectations for sharing feelings. Most people don't change their styles of communicating quickly. Measure your success in small steps.

Checking on results

Every week or so you should take time to think about how you are doing as a caregiver. Look through this home care plan and ask yourself how closely you are matching the "successful caregiver" that is described at the beginning of this plan.

If your plan doesn't work

Be realistic about what you expect of yourself. Don't expect to be perfect. Everyone makes mistakes. It takes time to learn to be a caregiver for someone with cancer. If there are some parts of caregiving that are especially difficult for you, then ask others for help.

If you cannot do the things that are essential for the person you are helping, then talk to the doctor, nurse, or social worker about getting the help that you need.

If you become so upset that it interferes with your ability to do what needs to be done or if you are having severe depression or anxiety symptoms (see the home care plans for Coping with Anxiety and Coping with Depression), then talk to the doctor, nurse, or social worker about getting help.

Fever and Infections

Overview of the
Home Care Plan for Fever and Infections

Understanding the Problem

       Why people receiving cancer treatments are at risk

       What the signs of infection are

       Fever as one sign of possible infection

When To Get Professional Help

       Symptoms and situations that require professional help because of emergency

       Symptoms and situations that require professional help during regular office hours

       Facts to know when you call for help

       What to say when you call

What You Can Do To Help

       Reduce fever after reporting it

       Prevent fever and infections

Possible Obstacles

       "High fevers burn up what is causing the problem."

       "Fevers will go away by themselves."

Carrying Out and Adjusting Your Plan

       Keep track of how frequently fevers occur

       Check to be sure that risky situations are avoided

       Report to medical staff if problems continue

(Topics with an arrow in front of them are actions you can take or symptoms you can look for.)

Fever and Infections

[The information in this home care plan fits most situations, but yours may be different.

If the doctor or nurse tells you to do something else, follow what they say. If you think there may be a medical emergency, see pages 25–26.]

Understanding the Problem

A person receiving chemotherapy or radiotherapy may be more likely to get infections. For a short time, chemotherapy or radiotherapy may reduce the white blood cell count, which leaves the person at a higher risk of infection. This condition is called neutropenia.

If signs of infection such as swelling, pain, or redness occur when the white blood cell count is low, it is important to treat the cause of these problems immediately. <u>Take action before a high temperature develops.</u> The body cannot fight infection when the number of white blood cells is low—early action is the key.

Fever is another sign of a possible infection. Fevers can be tiring, and the chills that may come with fevers can be frightening and exhausting. <u>A very high fever can also be dangerous</u>. Antibiotic medicines are often needed, at least until the number of white blood cells is back to normal.

Your goals are to:

call for help if it is needed,

lower fevers after reporting them, and

reduce the chance of future fevers and infections.

When To Get Professional Help

In case of an emergency

<u>Call the doctor, nurse, or the after-hours telephone number right away (no matter what time it is) if any of the following conditions exist</u>:

➤ **A temperature of 100.4 °F or higher by mouth.** Take the temperature if signs or symptoms of a cold or infection occur. A temperature of 98.6 °F is normal. Any higher number is a fever. Temperatures of 100.4 °F and higher usually indicate a problem requiring medical help.

Buy a new thermometer if you have one you don't trust or can't read. A digital thermometer is the easiest to use. It lights up and shows you the exact temperature when it is finished recording. Digital thermometers take the guess work out of deciding if a person has a fever. Ask your pharmacist or a store clerk to help you select one. Don't use a rectal thermometer unless your doctor or nurse approves its use. If the platelet count is low, the delicate tissue in the rectum may bleed when a thermometer is inserted.

➤ **A temperature 2 degrees higher than the person's normal temperature.** Ask the doctor or nurse what temperature indicates a fever for the person you are helping. Most normal oral temperatures are around 98.6 °F, but some people have normal temperatures that are higher or lower.

➤ **Severe shaking chills that last 20 minutes.** Chills occur before a temperature rises. Take the temperature when the chills are over and the shaking has stopped.

➤ **Frequent, painful urination.** Pain with urination usually indicates a urinary infection. People with this type of infection urinate in very small amounts. They also feel the urge to urinate even though little urine is in the bladder. When they do urinate, a sharp pain shoots through the lower abdomen.

➤ **No urine output for 6 to 8 hours.** It's important to report if the person has not urinated in the past day. This condition has many different possible causes and needs to be investigated.

➤ **New cough, shortness of breath, or rapid breathing.** Report any problems with breathing or coughing, especially a feeling that it is hard to draw air into the lungs or to release air. Labored or difficult breathing, with or without a fever, is important to report.

When symptoms are not an emergency, but should be reported

Some symptoms are not an emergency but should be reported during regular office or clinic hours. Call if any of the following conditions exist:

➤ **Too weak to drink fluids.** Drinking fluids is important. When the person's temperature rises, the body loses water which needs to be replaced. If it is not replaced, the person may become dehydrated. Fevers may cause severe fatigue, which makes it hard to drink. Therefore, when you report a fever, tell how much liquid the person has been drinking.

➤ **Any new redness or swelling on the skin or at an intravenous (IV) or injection site.** Skin redness or swelling may also indicate an infection. When the white blood cell counts are low, small cuts or scrapes can easily become infected.

➤ **Cold symptoms (runny nose, stuffy nose, watery eyes) or sore throat.** Infections develop quickly in the mouth or throat. Report cold symptoms, even when there is no fever.

➤ **New abdominal or back pain.** New pains in these areas may be the result of a new infection or the spread of an old infection.

➤ **Toothache.** Abscesses in the mouth or infected gums can cause toothaches. Antibiotics are often prescribed to prevent infection around the tooth. Dental work should be postponed until enough antibiotics are in the bloodstream to fight infection. Check with the doctor treating the infection before having any invasive dental work done.

Know the following facts before calling the doctor or nurse

How many hours has the fever been higher than 100.4 °F (by mouth)?

You may not know exactly how long the temperature has been high. Report the time that you took the temperature and the time that you first noticed any other changes, such as redder skin, more sweating, or complaints about feeling hot or feverish.

How much liquid did the person with fever drink since the fever began?

Report the amount of fluids the person drank and the amount of urine passed. This informs the doctor or nurse if dehydration (not having enough water in the body) from fever is becoming serious.

How much liquid was taken in the last 8 hours?

Has the person with cancer had other fevers since cancer treatments began? How many fevers? When have they occurred? After how many chemotherapy or radiation treatments did they begin?

If you know the pattern of past fevers after chemotherapy, give this information when you call. Some drugs create mild reactions for a short time. The doctor or nurse can judge what is normal for the drugs that were given.

What medicines were given to lower fever or fight infections (for example, acetaminophen [Tylenol™] or antibiotics)? When were they last taken?

When was the last chemotherapy treatment, and what were the names of the drugs given?

What were the most recent blood counts, and what date were the blood samples drawn?

Reporting this helps the doctor and nurse decide what may be causing the temperature and other symptoms. As a member of the health care team, your sharing of information is the key to treating a problem such as fever or infection successfully and quickly.

Here is an example of what you might say when calling about a fever or infection

"I am Joan Smith, Harry Smith's wife. My husband is Dr. Harvey's patient. The home care guide for fever says that I should call if shaking chills last over 20 minutes. They have. Then I took his temperature, and it was 101.6 °F. He had chemo last week. What should I do?"

What You Can Do To Help

There are two things you can do at home to deal with the problem of fever:

reduce the fever after reporting it, and

prevent fever and infection.

Reduce the fever after reporting it

Certain medicines (antipyretics) lower fevers. These drugs do not remove what caused the fever, but they do help lower the temperature and make the person feel better.

➤ **Give acetaminophen (adult dose) unless you have been told not to give it.** Acetaminophen (Tylenol™ and other brands) lowers body temperature. It also fights swelling and soreness and makes the person with cancer feel more comfortable. Acetaminophen does not make fever disappear, but it lowers the temperature and reduces the side effects of fever such as fatigue or aching.

➤ **Give any medications prescribed for fever or infection** by your doctor.

➤ **If the person with cancer is hot, put cold washcloths on the forehead.** Cooling the forehead brings some relief from the discomfort of feeling very hot. In addition, the cool cloths also cool the blood that flows through the head close to the surface of the skin.

➤ **Encourage the person to drink 2 to 3 quarts of cool liquid over 12 hours, unless large amounts of fluid are not allowed.** The body needs more fluid when feverish because more fluids than usual are being lost through the skin and lungs. The person with fever runs the risk of dehydration when the fever is high. Drinking fluids replaces lost water.

➤ **Serve high-calorie, high-carbohydrate foods.** The body's metabolism increases with fever. An increased metabolism means that the person with fever is burning calories at a faster rate than normal and so loses energy rapidly. High-calorie, high-carbohydrate foods replace the nutrients that are being burned up and help to restore some of the lost energy. Examples of these foods are pasta, bread, fruit, and potatoes.

➤ **Change damp clothing and bed linens.** When the person with fever sweats, moisture dries on the skin. This adds to discomfort and can also make the body cool down rapidly, causing shaking and chills.

Prevent fever and infection

Infections caught from others can be prevented by a combination of strategies. Here are some strategies to follow:

➤ **Don't share unwashed thermometers or toothbrushes.** Anything that goes in the mouth should not be shared because it's easy to pass germs from one person to another in this way.

➤ **Don't share drinking glasses.**

➤ **Avoid taking rectal temperatures.** These cannot be compared to oral temperatures, which are the ones usually recorded on the medical chart. Also, taking a rectal temperature adds to the risk of infection because the thermometer may cut or injure membranes inside the rectum. If it is not possible to obtain an oral temperature, place the thermometer under the person's armpit. This is known as axillary temperature.

➤ **Ask people with colds or who are ill to wait to visit** until they are better. Ask others to wait to visit until a cold is over. This lowers the risk of catching the cold and getting a fever.

➤ **Wash hands frequently,** especially before preparing food, before eating, and after using the bathroom.

➤ **Have the person with cancer wash frequently.** Hand washing is the best way to limit the spread of germs. People with cancer can get infections from their own skin, mouth, and tissues. They can also get infections from others. Wash the skin and hands frequently and brush the teeth at least three times a day to wash away potentially dangerous germs.

➤**Avoid raw fruit and vegetables that aren't washed, raw or undercooked eggs, and food handled by others,** only when the white blood cell count is low. Washing (or cooking) fruits and vegetables before eating them cleans off many germs. Deli items, which are already sliced, cannot usually be washed, so it's wise to buy and slice meats and cheeses yourself until white cell counts are higher and the risk of infection is lower. People with low white cell counts have difficulty warding off infections caught from others, and food is a common carrier of germs from other people.

➤**Offer liquids to prevent urinary infections.** Urinary infections are less likely to happen when the kidneys, bladder, and urinary system are flushed with water. Avoid caffeine and alcohol because these irritate the opening where the urine comes out and can break open the skin in that area.

➤**Replace toothbrushes every 3 months.** Toothbrushes harbor bacteria and other organisms because they are wet most of the time. Replace them as often as every 3 months to reduce the chance of infection in the mouth. New brushes are free of bacteria.

➤**Get a new toothbrush after treating a mouth infection** (usually a thrush infection).

➤**Encourage good dental hygiene,** including tooth brushing after eating and soaking dentures daily.

➤**Thoroughly clean the rectal area after bowel movements.** Women should cleanse the rectal area from front to back. This motion is less likely to cause a urinary infection because you are wiping away from the opening where urine comes out.

➤**Use sanitary pads and not tampons** during menstrual periods. Tampons breed bacteria more easily and can cause tears in the vagina that lead to infection.

➤**Thoroughly wash skin that is not open to the air,** such as the skin in the groin area and underneath the breasts.

➤**Wear shoes to prevent cuts and bruises.** Even small cuts on the feet can allow bacteria into the body. Cuts do not heal quickly when the white blood cell count is low.

➤**Wash cuts right away** with soap and water.

➤**Use a sunscreen lotion and stay out of the sun between 10:00 am and 3:00 pm.** Sunburn leads to blisters and splits the skin open. Once the skin is open, it's easier for bacteria to enter the body.

➤ **Use lotions and moisturizers** on the skin to prevent drying, chapping and cracking. Lotion keeps the skin moist and prevents dryness or cracking. Bacteria can enter dry skin cracks and start an infection.

➤ **Arrange for someone else to groom pets, empty cat litter boxes, and clean pet cages.** Pet feces contain many bacteria and fungi, which are easily transferred to a person with a low white blood cell count. It is best to have someone else clean the pets until the white blood cell count of the person with cancer returns to a normal level.

Possible Obstacles

Here are some obstacles that other people have faced

1. "High fevers burn up whatever is causing the problem."

   Response: <u>High fevers are dangerous</u> and should be reported and taken care of. If they are not, the temperature rises, and this body heat causes blood vessels to enlarge as they try to shed the heat. Water escapes through skin pores and through the lungs. Also, brain cells become more excitable because the body and its tissues are very hot. These two conditions can lead to dehydration and seizures. High temperatures do not burn up the bacteria that are causing the problem.

2. "I've had fevers before, and they didn't last long. It will go away by itself."

   Response: Fevers can be serious and should be reported and treated. If they are not, the temperature may rise too high and may lead to dehydration. <u>Avoid high temperatures and report any possible signs of infection whether or not a fever occurs with them</u>. When the white blood cell count is low, fevers will not disappear on their own.

Think of *other* obstacles that could interfere with carrying out your plan

What additional road blocks could get in the way of doing the things recommended in this home care plan? For example, will the person with cancer cooperate? Will other people help? How will you explain your needs to other people? Do you have the time and energy to carry out the plan?

You need to develop plans for getting around these road blocks. Use the four COPE ideas (creativity, optimism, planning, and expert information) in developing your plans. See the chapter on Solving Home Care Problems at the beginning of the book for a discussion of how to use the four COPE ideas in overcoming your obstacles.

Carrying Out and Adjusting Your Plan

Checking on results

Keep records of when fevers happen so that you can see if they are occurring more or less often. Check regularly to <u>be sure that the person with cancer is avoiding situations that increase the risk of his or her getting an infection</u>.

If your plan doesn't work

If fever remains a problem, if your plan does not seem to be working, or if fevers are happening more often, there are two things you can do. Consider them in this order:

1. Check the section titled When To Get Professional Help in this home care plan. If you answer "yes" to any of those questions, call the doctor or nurse immediately.

2. <u>If fever problems continue, ask the doctor or nurse for help</u>. Tell them what you have done and what the results have been.

Tiredness and Fatigue

Overview of the
Home Care Plan for Tiredness and Fatigue

Understanding the Problem

Reasons why people with cancer feel tired

Let the person with cancer decide how much he or she can do

When To Get Professional Help

Symptoms that require professional help immediately

Symptoms that should be reported during regular office hours

Facts to know when you call for help

What to say when you call

What You Can Do To Help

Help the person get the most out of the day

Promote rest and sleep

Possible Obstacles

"There's nothing we can do about it."

"Worry keeps him/her awake."

Carrying Out and Adjusting Your Plan

Keep track of sleep

Decide if he or she is using awake time well

Report problems to medical staff

(Topics with an arrow in front of them are actions you can take or symptoms you can look for.)

Tiredness and Fatigue

[The information in this home care plan fits most situations, but yours may be different.

If the doctor or nurse tells you to do something else, follow what they say. If you think there may be a medical emergency, see page 36.]

Understanding the Problem

People with cancer can feel very worn out and tired. Tiredness may be caused by the disease itself or by the treatments. It may be caused by anemia, which means there are fewer red blood cells circulating oxygen to the body. Anemia can be caused by cancer, chemotherapy, or nutritional problems and can be prevented or decreased by taking iron pills, vitamin B_{12} folate, or drugs that stimulate the production of red blood cells. These drugs (human erythropoietin) can improve energy and activity levels and reduce the need for blood transfusions.

Other causes of tiredness are malnutrition (not eating enough) or a temporary increase in waste products as cancer cells are destroyed by radiation therapy or chemotherapy.

Sometimes people feel tired after each course of treatment for their cancer. They complain of not having enough energy or not feeling like they can get going.

Tiredness also may happen because normal resting and sleep habits are disrupted. It may happen because the person with cancer is feeling depressed or in pain.

You should not "push" the person with cancer to do more than what she or he feels is reasonable. Let him or her decide how much to do. If other symptoms occur with increased fatigue, then it's important to talk with the doctor or nurse.

Your goals are for the person with cancer to:

have as little tiredness as possible,

use energy as effectively as possible, and

keep regular schedules of sleep and rest.

When To Get Professional Help

Tiredness, by itself, is not an emergency. However, some other symptoms that may occur in combination with tiredness are serious. When these symptoms occur, you should get immediate help.

In case of an emergency

Call the doctor or nurse if any of the following conditions exist in addition to tiredness:

➤ **Severe or frequent dizziness.** Dizziness, or feeling a loss of balance, can happen when walking, getting out of bed, or going from a standing to a sitting position. Dizziness can also occur without moving or changing one's position. This symptom can happen to anyone occasionally. When it is severe and frequent, you should get medical help.

➤ **Falling followed by an injury, bleeding, mental confusion, or unconsciousness.** Report all bad falls so the doctor or nurse can judge what caused the fall, whether bones were broken, and what follow-up is needed. Sometimes they'll recommend using equipment for safety reasons. For example, canes, walkers, or bedside commodes can be helpful to people who feel extremely tired.

➤ **Inability to wake up.** You should call right away if you cannot wake up the person with cancer or if a sudden and unexpected change in the level of consciousness or alertness occurs. You will probably have to take the person to a medical facility for tests to determine the cause of this problem.

➤ **Feeling out of breath.** Breathlessness usually happens because the body is not getting the right amount of air and oxygen. This can be caused by a problem with the lungs and respiratory system or by a low level of red blood cells.

When symptoms are not an emergency, but should be reported

Other problems that might appear with fatigue that should also be reported during regular office or clinic hours are:

➤ **Ringing in the ears.** This problem could be caused by a reaction to medication, a change in blood flow to the brain, or other physical problems. Medical tests are usually required to determine its cause.

➤ **Pounding in the head.** This problem can also signal a problem with blood flow or blood pressure. Medical tests are usually required to determine its cause.

➤ **Staying in bed for days.** Staying in bed can be a sign of depression if it continues for days on end without other symptoms. See the home care plan for Coping with Depression if this happens. Not getting out of bed can also be caused by fatigue, in which case treatment for anemia may restore some energy.

Know the following facts before you call the doctor or nurse

1. How clear are his or her thoughts compared with the person's thoughts before the symptoms happened?

2. Has any confusion appeared or increased since fatigue increased?

3. Is the person with cancer feeling depressed or "blue"?

4. Has any new medicine been started, such as pain medicine or sleep medicine?

Here is an example of what you might say when calling

"I am Joan Smith, Harry Smith's wife. My husband is Dr. Harvey's patient. The home care plan for fatigue says that I should call if he feels some pounding in his head. He's been very tired lately, and today he complained of this pounding. He says it feels different from a headache."

What You Can Do To Help

If you decide that tiredness is not an emergency, there are two things you can do to help solve this problem:

help the person get the most out of the day, and

promote rest and sleep.

Help the person get the most out of the day

➤ **Plan the day so that being with people or trips happen when he or she feels most refreshed and awake.** Plan activities during the time of day when the person feels best. Allow time for rest between events.

➤ **Rest between bathing, dressing, and walking.**

➤ **Conserve energy by doing things only for a short time.** Schedule activities in parts that can be done for a short time. Also encourage resting ahead of time.

➤ **Agree on what's most important to do.** Discuss which activities bring the most enjoyment or are necessary. Start with the most necessary or enjoyable activities, and don't be disappointed if all things on the list do not get done.

➤ **Avoid dizziness or falls by getting up or moving slowly.** Avoid dizziness with normal movement. Dizziness can result from fatigue. When persons with cancer get up from lying down, remind them to sit on the bedside and dangle the feet and legs for at least 4 minutes before standing up.

➤ **Plan regular exercise to reduce fatigue.** Plan something to do every day despite the fatigue, even if it's as little as getting dressed or walking out to sit on the porch. Short walks are also helpful.

➤ **Serve snacks as well as regular meals.** Add liver and red meat to the diet because of needed proteins and iron. Serve a well-balanced diet from the four food groups (dairy, fruit and vegetables, breads and cereals, and proteins such as meat, chicken, fish, or eggs). Ask family and neighbors to bring food, or call a community meals program to deliver balanced meals. They have meals for people on low-sodium and diabetic diets, if needed. The most important food group is nutritious carbohydrates, which give the most energy. Examples of carbohydrates are pasta, bread, fruit, and potatoes.

Promote rest and sleep

➤ **Keep as active as possible during the day so that normal fatigue sets in at night.** If the person with cancer remains active throughout the day, then sleep is easier at night.

➤ **Resume usual patterns of rest and sleep** as much as possible. Set regular times to nap and sleep, which helps the person's body come to expect a routine. Routine habits help sleep.

➤ **Read the home care plan for Coping with Anxiety if nervousness or anxiety interrupts rest or sleep.** The plan has some good ideas on handling anxiety, including instructions on how to become relaxed. Talking with, touching, and listening to the person can also help manage anxiety.

➤ **Encourage rest when tired by going to bed earlier, sleeping later, and taking naps during the day.** If naps are a habit, then taking longer ones allows more rest and helps to reduce fatigue.

➤ **Play relaxing music before sleep.** Use whatever helped to promote sleep before. Music or the sound of the television or of someone reading can be very soothing.

➤ **Meditation or prayer before bedtime can also help a person to fall asleep.**

➤ **Drink warm milk at bedtime.**

➤ **Give a warm bath or back rub at bedtime.**

➤ **Try sleeping pills.** If you have done the above things on this list and the person with cancer still is having trouble sleeping, ask the doctor if sleeping medicine would help. Do not give sleeping medicine without checking with the doctor. These medicines can cause problems when combined with other drugs. Be sure that the physician is aware of all other medicines being taken when you ask about sleeping pills.

Possible Obstacles

Here are some obstacles that have interfered with other people's plans for dealing with tiredness and fatigue

1. "The fatigue comes with the treatments. There's nothing we can do to help it."

   Response: Cancer treatments often do result in fatigue, but <u>you can control how tiredness affects your life</u>. Many things can be tried to help reduce a feeling of fatigue, including new medicines to prevent anemia (low red blood cell counts).

2. "There are so many things to worry about. No wonder I can't sleep."

   Response: <u>Sleep helps to reduce some of the anxiety</u> because physical fatigue can add to feeling anxious and jumpy. Set a goal of better rest as one of your top priorities.

Think of *other* obstacles that could interfere with carrying out your plan

What additional road blocks could get in the way of doing the things recommended in this home care plan? For example, will the person with cancer cooperate? Will other people help? How will you explain your needs to other people? Do you have the time and energy to carry out the plan?

You will need to develop plans for getting around these road blocks. Use the four COPE ideas (creativity, optimism, planning, and expert information) in developing your plans. See the chapter on Solving Home Care Problems at the beginning of the book for a discussion of how to use the four COPE ideas in overcoming your obstacles.

Carrying Out and Adjusting Your Plan

Checking on results

Keep track of how much of the day the person with cancer spends in bed. <u>Ask the person to prioritize activities and choose those that are important and rewarding</u>. Check on whether current patterns of sleep and rest are similar to patterns before the illness.

If your plan doesn't work

If your plan doesn't seem to be working, ask yourself if you are expecting change too fast. It usually takes time to work out ways to live with tiredness.

<u>If tiredness is increasing and is of major concern to the person with cancer, ask the doctor or nurse for help</u>. Tell them what you have done and what the results have been.

Problems with Appetite

Overview of the
Home Care Plan for Problems with Appetite

Understanding the Problem

Why appetite is lost

Weight loss can be slowed by stopping diarrhea, giving high-calorie foods, or taking medicines that stimulate appetite

When To Get Professional Help

Situations and symptoms that require professional help

Facts to know when you call for help

What to say

What You Can Do To Help

Increase the appetite

Cover up tastes or smells

Prevent an early feeling of fullness

Add more proteins and calories to food

Possible Obstacles

"I'm not interested in food."

"Why bother with adding calories to food?"

Carrying Out and Adjusting Your Plan

Keep track of foods and fluids

Talk to nurse or dietician for other ideas

(Topics with an arrow in front of them are actions you can take or symptoms you can look for.)

Problems with Appetite

[The information in this home care plan fits most situations, but yours may be different.

If the doctor or nurse tells you to do something else, follow what they say. If you think there may be a medical emergency, see pages 43–44.]

Understanding the Problem

People with cancer lose their appetite for many reasons. Cancer treatments and other medicines can decrease the desire for food, as can emotional distress or worry.

Losing weight can upset the person with cancer especially if he or she sees it as a sign that the illness is getting worse. Rapid weight loss, however, can often be slowed down by stopping diarrhea, giving high-calorie foods, or taking medicines prescribed to help the appetite.

This home care plan describes the things you can do to help increase appetite. In addition, many booklets are available on eating problems during cancer treatment, including some with recipes, produced by the National Cancer Institute and the American Cancer Society and by companies that manufacture dietary supplements. Physicians who treat persons with cancer often keep a supply of these booklets in their offices.

Your goals are to:

call for professional help when it is needed,

encourage ways to increase the appetite,

cover up tastes and smells that are bothersome,

prevent an early feeling of fullness, and

add more proteins and calories to what is eaten.

When To Get Professional Help

The first question you should ask is whether professional help is needed. Show this home care plan to the doctor or nurse and have them fill in the blanks. Then call if any of the following conditions exist:

➤ **The person has had very little to eat or drink in ___ days.** Ask the doctor or nurse when you should report a poor appetite. If nausea causes the loss of appetite, then read the home care plan on nausea for steps you can take to relieve that symptom. When nausea lasts more than a few days and little is eaten, it's important to keep the doctor or nurse informed so that the situation doesn't develop into an emergency.

➤ **___ pounds are lost in one week**. <u>Ask the doctor or nurse when to call about weight loss</u>. If the person with cancer is losing weight, then talk about this on a clinic visit or with the home health nurses if they are visiting the home.

➤ **There is pain with chewing or swallowing**. Painful chewing or swallowing interferes with normal eating and drinking. Pain can be caused by a mouth sore or an infection on the tongue, gums, or throat. If the appetite suddenly changes, ask the person if he or she is having trouble eating, chewing, or swallowing.

Know the following facts before you call the doctor or nurse

1. When did the poor appetite problem start?
2. If this problem happened before, what brought the appetite back or helped it improve?
3. Does food taste differently, for example, bitter or metallic? If so, does this make foods less desirable?
4. Which foods taste better than they used to and which taste worse?
5. Is the person's mouth dry or sore and is swallowing difficult?
6. Do you have medication to help with mouth problems?
7. Does the person feel full or bloated soon after starting to eat?
8. Is the person having nausea, vomiting, or problems with bowels such as constipation or diarrhea? If so, what medicines are available for these problems in the home and which of these have you tried for this problem?
9. When the appetite changed, was there a change in where or how food was eaten?
10. Does the person have a better or worse appetite at certain meals or certain times of day?
11. How much weight has been lost?

Here is an example of what you might say when calling for help

"I am Mary Smith, Harry Smith's wife. My husband is Dr. Harvey's patient. The home care plan for appetite says that we should call if he complains of a sore mouth. It's so sore that he's having trouble chewing."

What You Can Do To Help

There are four approaches you can use to solve problems with appetite:

increase the appetite,

cover up tastes or smells,

prevent an early feeling of fullness, and

add more protein and calories to food.

Increase the appetite

Sometimes people with cancer lose their appetite because of treatments or emotional distress. <u>There are several things you can do to help stimulate appetite</u>:

➤ **Encourage light exercise or walking before meals,** in fresh air if possible. Any increase in activity just before eating increases the appetite. Try walking 5 to 15 minutes or up to half an hour before meals. Fresh air always stimulates the appetite.

➤ **Serve meals with other people,** whenever possible. Avoid eating alone. Eating with someone else is distracting and can increase the amount a person eats by taking attention away from food. Sometimes meal habits change after a diagnosis of cancer because the person doesn't feel like eating or the family schedule is disrupted by trips to clinics for checkups and treatments. Returning to normal meal times and planning to have the family eat together helps to increase the appetite.

➤ **Serve meals nicely in a pleasant, relaxed atmosphere,** if possible.

➤ **Use small plates and serve smaller portions.** A small portion on a small plate can be arranged attractively and looks like something that can be finished.

➤ **Keep food out of sight when not eating.** Keep food off counter tops and put it in containers that you can't see through. Then the person with cancer is not reminded about the appetite problem by seeing food all of the time. As a result, food may be more appealing when served.

➤ **Serve lemonade or orange juice if the mouth is not sore.** Juices contain acids which can stimulate appetites. Four ounces before a meal may improve the appetite.

➤ **Serve a glass of wine or beer or a cocktail before lunch or dinner, if the doctor approves.** Alcohol stimulates the appetite. Alcohol should not be taken, however, with certain medications and should not be taken before chemotherapy treatments because it can cause nausea and even change the effect of the drugs. It can weaken the strength of a medicine or make it too powerful. Consult your physician and pharmacist about alcohol limits or about drinking at all. It is not allowed during chemotherapy.

Cover up tastes and smells that are bothersome

Cancer treatments frequently change how foods taste. There are a number of things you can do to make food appealing again:

➤ **Use plastic utensils.** They take away a bitter or metal taste, which is a common complaint among persons receiving chemotherapy.

➤ **Try new spices,** such as basil, curry, coriander, mint, oregano, or rosemary. Spices make our mouths water and change the tastes of food. You may find a new spice that makes the person hungry again. Try old spices in new ways because the chemotherapy sometimes changes the way food tastes.

➤ **Add new flavors,** such as lemon, beer, pickles, salad dressings, vinegar, mayonnaise, relishes, fruit juices, or wines.

➤ **Marinate meats** in liquids, such as fruit juices, salad dressings, wine, sweet and sour sauce, soy sauce, or barbecue sauce. Sauces and marinades change the flavor of food and make it more appealing.

➤ **Sprinkle more sugar and salt in food if these are not restricted.** These decrease the metal and bitter tastes that persons with cancer sometimes complain about. Some people receiving chemotherapy cannot tolerate a sweet taste, in which case you should use smaller amounts of sugar than before.

➤ **Choose nutritious carbohydrates and high-protein options,** such as fish, chicken, turkey, eggs, cheeses, milk, ice cream, tofu, nuts, peanut butter, yogurt, beans, or peas. Try to get as much protein and carbohydrate as possible from each food item served. This is called "power-packing" foods.

➤ **Eat food cold.** A cold temperature downplays the smell and taste of food. Aromas are blocked or linger for shorter times, and cold foods are not as flavorful so that odd tastes are covered up. Also the coolness numbs the tongue to some unpleasant tastes.

➤ **Suck on hard, sugar-free, sour, or mint candy.** Candies like these can mask strange tastes any time of the day and even before a meal.

➤ **Drink ginger ale or mint tea.** They cover up metallic tastes and help with swallowing food.

> **Avoid most red meats and eat chicken, fish, or pork.** Changes in taste buds may make red meat distasteful. People receiving chemotherapy often prefer chicken or fish, which retain their flavors.

Prevent an early feeling of fullness

Poor appetite can be caused by an early feeling of being full. Sometimes medicines cause gas, and the person feels bloated after eating very little. Following are six things that can be done to deal with this problem:

> **Exercise between meals.** Any exercise gets the intestinal tract moving and shakes up pockets of gas. Even stretching and bending the waist by getting out of chairs or off of couches helps relieve gas and move stomach contents downward.

> **Walk around or sit up for awhile after meals, but avoid strenuous exercise immediately after eating.** This action helps to empty the stomach and break up any gas that adds to a sense of fullness and discomfort.

> **Drink beverages between meals instead of with meals.** Liquids at mealtime can make the stomach feel full. Drinking less while eating allows more room for food.

> **Eat small amounts of food 6 to 8 times a day.** Small, frequent meals or snacks prevent an early sense of fullness, and more food can be eaten over a 24-hour period.

> **Eat slowly and chew food well.**

> **Avoid certain vegetables and carbonation.** Cut back on fatty foods and gas-producing foods such as beans, cucumbers, green peppers, onions, broccoli, brussel sprouts, corn, cauliflower, sauerkraut, turnips, cabbage, chewing gum, milk, rutabagas, or carbonated beverages. Some vegetables naturally create stomach and intestinal gas and keep the person with cancer feeling full as the food is slowly digested. Avoid these items as well as carbonated sodas or waters. Remove the carbonation by opening cans and bottles early and letting the fizz evaporate and the sodas turn flat.

> **Use over-the-counter medicines to help break up gas.** Many of these medicines contain herbs or drugs that break up gas. One particular ingredient, simethicone, is helpful in attacking gas and breaking up air trapped in the intestines. Check with the doctor and nurse before buying these over-the-counter medicines because they shouldn't be used with some other medicines.

Add more proteins and calories to food

Rapid weight loss can often be slowed by increasing the nutritional value of food that is eaten, especially by increasing the calories and proteins. Here are some suggestions for how you can make the food that is eaten count more toward keeping on weight.

➤ **Offer small, frequent snacks (six per day) even if the person is not hungry, and encourage eating as much as wanted.** Smaller meals and snacks may add up to a higher protein and calorie intake in a 24-hour period.

➤ **Add butter or margarine to vegetables, soups, pasta, cooked cereal, and rice.** These add fat and calories and improve the taste of many foods.

➤ **Add sugar, syrup, honey, and jelly to vegetables, meats, cereals, waffles, and rolls.** Sweet sauces add calories and can make dry foods easier to swallow.

➤ **Use sour cream or cream cheese on baked potatoes, vegetables, and crackers.** Creams are fattening, nutritious, and easy to swallow. Use them to add many more calories to the diet.

➤ **Add whipped cream to hot chocolate, ice cream, pies, puddings, gelatin, and other desserts.** Whipped cream is loaded with calories. Add sugar to whipped cream and boost calories even higher.

➤ **Add powdered coffee creamers or powdered milk to gravy, sauces, soups, and hot cereals.** These are good sources of calcium and increase the number of calories in food without adding bulk.

➤ **Use milk instead of water to dilute condensed soups or cooked cereals.** If a recipe calls for water, use milk instead. This will add calories and important nutrients and vitamins.

➤ **Use mayonnaise instead of salad dressing and use light cream instead of milk** in recipes. Mayonnaise and light cream have more fat and calories than salad dressing and milk. Avoid skim milk, if possible.

➤ **Add ice cream to milk drinks.** Ice cream increases the fat and calorie content in milk and feels good on sore throats.

➤ **Add nonfat dry milk (1 cup) to 1 quart of whole milk for drinking and cooking.** You can more than double the protein and calorie content of regular (4%) milk if you add powdered dry milk to it.

➤ **Use half-and-half or evaporated milk instead of water in recipes.** Half cream and half milk or evaporated milk are much higher in fat, protein, and calories than water. They also provide vital minerals and nutrients. Many people with cancer drink "instant breakfast" mixes for extra calories. These are sold in grocery stores.

➤ **Use peanut butter** on crackers, bread, waffles, apple wedges, or celery sticks. Peanut butter is an excellent source of protein.

➤ **Offer crushed granola, nuts, seeds, or wheat germ in shakes or on desserts.**

➤ **Use nutritional supplements such as Isocal™, Ensure™, Sustacal™, Resource™, or Citrotein™ between meals or with snacks.** These powders or liquids are loaded with nutrients and can be purchased in most drug stores. Ask the nurse or pharmacist for information about buying them and ask for recipes. Also, in some states, the American Cancer Society will purchase these supplements for you, if you cannot pay for them.

➤ **Avoid diets designed to "purge the system."** Certain diets are designed to purge or empty the intestinal tract. Unfortunately, they also remove important vitamins, minerals, and fluids from the body. The person with cancer needs these nutrients.

➤ **Ask the nurse or doctor about using vitamin supplements and iron.** Vitamin supplements replace some vitamins lost because of a smaller appetite and smaller intake of food. The doctor or nurse may suggest daily multivitamin and iron pills as supplements to the diet.

Possible Obstacles

Here are some obstacles that other caregivers have faced when trying to solve appetite problems

1. "He says he's just not interested in food. He's not hungry at all."

   Response: Lack of interest in food cannot be easily changed. <u>Try to offer small snacks or meals in the company of people he or she enjoys</u>. Try the other suggestions in this home care plan, but don't focus on eating so much so that it's the only topic you ask about or talk about.

2. "Why bother with adding calories to food? The treatments will make her so sick that she won't eat anyway."

> Response: Cancer treatments do not cause as much nausea as they used to. New drugs to prevent nausea are very good now. Adding calories to food helps to prevent anemia and increase energy. It will also help keep weight on. All of these benefits help the person with cancer to handle the cancer treatments and feel better.

Think of *other* obstacles that could interfere with carrying out your plan

What additional road blocks could get in the way of doing the things recommended in this home care plan? For example, will the person with cancer cooperate? Will other people help? How will you explain your needs to other people? Do you have the time and energy to carry out the plan?

You need to develop plans for getting around these road blocks. Use the four COPE ideas (creativity, optimism, planning, and expert information) in developing your plans. See the chapter on Solving Home Care Problems at the beginning of the book for a discussion of how to use the four COPE ideas in overcoming your obstacles.

Carrying Out and Adjusting Your Plan

Checking on results

Keep track of the amount of food the person with cancer is eating as well as his or her weight. If you find a problem, check to see if you should call the doctor or nurse. Ask the person with cancer if eating is being hindered by bothersome tastes and smells, dry or sore mouth, or an early feeling of fullness. If so, use the ideas in this home care plan.

If your plan doesn't work

If you are not satisfied with progress toward increasing appetite, talk about your concerns with the doctor or nurse. They may refer you to a dietician who will give you new ideas or who will tell you whether the diet is adequate and whether you are packing as many nutrients as you can into the foods you are serving. The doctor may also prescribe an appetite stimulant or make other suggestions to help you deal with this problem.

Problems with the Mouth

Overview of the
Home Care Plan for Problems with the Mouth

Understanding the Problem

Why people get mouth sores with chemotherapy

How mouth sores lead to infections

When To Get Professional Help

Symptoms that require professional help

Facts to know when you call for help

What to say when you call

What You Can Do To Help

Moisten a dry mouth

Soothe a sore mouth and ease swallowing

How to treat mouth sores, ulcers, or infections

How to prevent mouth sores

Possible Obstacles

"Who wants to quit smoking or drinking?"

"It's upsetting to have soft foods."

Carrying Out and Adjusting Your Plan

Follow a daily mouth care schedule

Check on how uncomfortable the mouth sores are

Check to see if they interfere with eating

Call the doctor or nurse if mouth sores do not heal

(Topics with an arrow in front of them are actions you can take or symptoms you can look for.)

Problems with the Mouth

[The information in this home care plan fits most situations, but yours may be different.

If the doctor or nurse tells you to do something else, follow what they say. If you think there may be a medical emergency, see pages 53–54.]

Understanding the Problem

<u>Problems with the mouth are a common side effect of cancer treatments</u> because the skin inside of the mouth is composed of rapidly growing cells. Chemotherapy can slow the growth of healthy cells in the mouth. As a result, the mouth tissues are weakened, mouth sores develop, and sores take longer to heal.

In addition, cancer and cancer treatments can temporarily reduce the ability of a person's immune system to fight infection. When the immune system cannot protect the body from normal bacteria or outside germs, weakened or inflamed tissues in the mouth can become infected. A sore and tender throat and esophagus can also develop.

Your goals are to:

call for help when it is needed,

treat mouth sores, ulcers, or infections, and

prevent mouth problems.

When To Get Professional Help

Report the signs and symptoms listed below to the doctor or nurse. They can then take steps to determine if an infection is beginning in the mouth, tongue, throat, or esophagus (the tube leading to the stomach). Sometimes these problems can become so severe that the person must take pain medication or be hospitalized for antibiotic therapy.

You should call the clinic, doctor, or nurse if any of the following conditions exist

➤ **Temperature over 100.4 °F.** Fever can indicate a mouth infection. If the temperature goes up suddenly, report it. However, a mouth infection can occur before the temperature goes up, so fever is not the only thing to watch for.

➤ **A light redness on the tongue gets *much* redder.** Redness comes before a mouth sore. You will need a light to tell if the mouth, gums, or tongue are redder than usual. Use a small flashlight to look into the mouth and find sores. Check the mouth twice a day, morning and night. Look at the roof of the mouth and all of the lining. Look under the tongue and gums.

➤ **Redness on tongue turns to white patches or white patches appear on gums or in mouth.** White patches indicate an infection. Usually it's a thrush infection (called *Candida albicans*). This infection occurs when the lining in the mouth is unable to fight off normal bacteria, and, as a result, bacteria increase in number and become a problem.

➤ **Complaint of "cotton" mouth or a very thick feeling on the tongue when rubbed against upper teeth.** A cottony feeling in the mouth or on the tongue also means that an infection may be starting. Call and report this right away.

➤ **Sore or ulcer on the lips or in the mouth.** If the normal skin covering the mouth is changed by chemotherapy, mouth soreness and sometimes mouth sores or ulcers follow.

➤ **Sore throat or painful throat.** The lining of the throat is the same as the lining of the mouth. The throat is just as likely to get red and sore as the mouth is.

➤ **So much difficulty swallowing that medicine is not being taken as often as prescribed.** Trouble with swallowing prevents taking medicine. When the throat is sore or swollen, swallowing becomes more difficult. Call if medicines are skipped because swallowing is too painful.

➤ **So much difficulty swallowing or drinking and eating that little food or fluid is taken for 2 days.** The person with cancer may be eating or drinking less because of a sore or painful throat. This can cause weakness and possibly dehydration. Treatment for mouth soreness will help with eating and drinking.

Know the following facts before you call the doctor or nurse

1. When did the mouth problems start?

2. Is the mouth, tongue, or throat redder than usual?

3. Are there white patches in the mouth?

4. What was eaten and how many liquids were taken in the past 48 hours?

5. How are the mouth and teeth cleaned? Are any special rinses used to prevent mouth sores?

6. Is the person with cancer smoking? If yes, how much?

7. Was any alcohol taken? If yes, how much?

8. Is there a change in chewing or swallowing?

9. Has any medicine been ordered for the mouth or throat? If so, how often is it taken?

10. Do any medicines for the mouth cause problems such as gagging or nausea when taken so that they are taken less often than prescribed?

11. When was the last radiation or chemotherapy treatment and what chemotherapy drugs were given?

Here is an example of what you might say when calling

"I am Joan Smith, Harry Smith's wife. My husband is Dr. Harvey's patient. The home care plan for mouth sores says that I should call if he has a cottony feeling in his mouth. Also, his throat hurts so badly that he is only taking the medicine once a day that was prescribed for 4 times a day."

What You Can Do To Help

If you do not need to call the doctor or nurse, here are four things you can do to help solve problems with mouth sores or a sore mouth:

moisten a dry mouth,

soothe a sore mouth and ease swallowing,

treat mouth sores, ulcers, or infections, and

prevent mouth problems.

Moisten a dry mouth

Dry mouth is a frequent side effect of medicines taken for cancer. A dry mouth makes it harder to chew and swallow. There are several things you can do to deal with dry mouth:

➤ **Rinse the mouth before meals and throughout the day.** Rinsing the mouth helps to moisten it and remove the feeling of being parched or dry, but don't use rinses that have alcohol in them because they dry the mouth.

➤ **Use a lip moisturizer before eating.** If the lips are moist, food is easier to chew and enjoy. Use petroleum jelly, lip salve, or cocoa butter.

➤ **Sip 2 to 3 quarts of liquid a day, unless large amounts of fluid are not allowed.**

➤ **Eat ice chips, Popsicles™, frozen juices, or frozen drinks.** They provide liquids and can be quite refreshing. The sugar content in Popsicles™ also makes the mouth water, which decreases dryness.

➤ **Drink small sips of liquids with meals.**

➤ **Dunk bread, crackers, and baked foods in coffee, tea, milk, or soup to make them moist.** Moistening food is another easy way to fight a dry mouth. Dip bread in soup, shredded meat in marinade, or toast in coffee.

➤ **Mix gravies, sauces, salad dressings, melted butter or margarine, mayonnaise, or yogurt into food.** Sauces and gravies go a long way to moisten food and make it easier to chew and swallow. They can be added toward the end of cooking or when food is reheated.

➤ **Serve soft, liquid foods** such as applesauce, canned fruits, casseroles, cooked cereal, baby foods, Popsicles™, custard, bananas, puddings, ice cream, gelatin, sherbet, yogurt, milk shakes, soups, stews, watermelon, and seedless grapes. If the food is not liquid to begin with, grind it or put it in a blender. Many people with cancer use blenders to enjoy foods that they cannot chew easily. Even a steak can be tenderized and pureed and all of the good flavor remains.

➤ **Ask about artificial saliva.** Bottles of artificial saliva can be ordered through most pharmacies. It comes in a bottle and is made of glycerin, purified water, and a few other ingredients. Xerolube™, Mouthkote™ or Salivert™ are examples of commercial products that are available in a mint flavor, and many people have found these products helpful in reducing problems with dry mouth.

Soothe a sore mouth and ease swallowing

Some chemotherapy causes mouth sores, which make eating and swallowing difficult. Here are things to do for this problem:

➤ **Rinse the mouth with baking soda after eating,** using a solution of 1/2 teaspoon of baking soda in 1 cup of tap water. Salt or baking soda, or both, soothes the mouth and helps it heal. Rinsing after eating removes food particles that could irritate the gums, but it does so more gently than commercial mouthwashes, many of which contain alcohol. Avoid mouthwashes with alcohol because they dry out the mouth.

➤ **Drink plenty of liquids and suck on ice chips.**

➤ **Use a blender or hand masher to soften foods.** Softer foods are easier to chew and swallow. They are less likely to tear any sores or scrape raw tissues.

➤ **Moisten food with cream, milk, gravy, and sauces.** Moist food is easier to swallow, especially when the mouth and throat are tender.

➤ **Drink pureed food from a cup or through a straw.** Soft food can be liquefied in a blender and poured into a cup for drinking. Using a straw helps the liquid bypass some of the sore mouth tissue when eating. Many proteins and calories can be taken in this way. If the person is too weak to use a straw, then fill the straw with an inch or two of liquid and drop the liquid in the mouth slowly.

➤ **Eat soft, moist, bland foods** such as soups, eggs, pastas, quiches, baby foods, cheese dishes, tuna fish, applesauce, custards, pudding, canned fruit, cooked cereals, bananas, gelatin, yogurt, ice cream, sherbet, frozen fruit bars, Popsicles™, or shakes. Bland foods are those that are not spicy or salty. Examples are bread, pudding, gelatin, custard, rice, and tapioca. All are soft, moist, and easier to swallow than other foods when the mouth or throat are easily irritated.

Treat mouth sores, ulcers, or infections

Use the following list at the first hint of a sore or infection to reduce the seriousness of mouth and throat complications.

➤ **Rinse the mouth with warm tap water after eating or drinking, or use any of these:**

1/2 teaspoon salt to 2 cups of water

1/2 teaspoon baking soda to 1 cup of water

1/2 teaspoon salt and 1/2 teaspoon baking soda to 2 cups of water

Mouth rinses remove food particles that may build up and cause bacteria to grow. Rinses also soothe sore tissues and help them heal faster. Rinse at least four times a day and as often as every 2 hours while awake, if possible. If the salt rinse burns, use the baking soda recipe or less salt.

➤ **Ask about using a numbing liquid to use as a "throat coat" before eating and swallowing.** Many people swallow mouth gels or "throat coats"™ (a thick jelly-like liquid) before meals and at bedtime when the mouth is very sore because of chemotherapy. This medicine numbs the tongue and throat enough to let liquid and soft foods pass without much trouble. The medicine also usually contains Maalox™ and liquid Benadryl™, which heal and soothe the soreness and decrease swelling and inflammation, especially in the throat and esophagus. Ask about these mouth gels or medicines if they haven't been prescribed as part of the chemotherapy.

Another type of soothing medicine (called a "slurry") comes in tablet form and dissolves in water. It works quickly to remove any burning feeling and helps to heal the lining of the mouth and throat. Report to the doctor if the person is having trouble swallowing liquid medicines for the mouth and not using them as often as prescribed. The doctor may order another type of mouth treatment.

➤ **Use a topical ointment on sores to soothe pain or soreness.** Some mouth sores cause so much pain that they prevent the person from eating and chewing. Coating the sores with a topical ointment numbs them long enough to help with eating.

➤ **Ask about prescription mouth rinses to swish and swallow.** During chemotherapy and a few weeks after treatment, many people use a prescription mouth rinse to swish and swallow at least four times per day. This prevents infection and eases soreness.

➤ **Finish liquid antibiotics when they are prescribed to treat an infection.** The doctor may also order an oral liquid antibiotic. If so, be sure that all of it is taken until the bottle is empty. Antibiotics are ordered to kill the mouth infection. If they are effective, the person's mouth should feel better and eating and drinking should be easier in a few days.

➤ **Ask about using mild pain pills.** Mild pain medicines can be taken an hour before eating and drinking. They help reduce the pain of biting, chewing, or swallowing when the mouth feels sore or when there are ulcers.

➤ **Avoid using peroxide or peroxide rinses.** Peroxide kills bacteria, but it is drying. Its use can lead to a mouth and throat infection known as thrush. In rare cases, a peroxide rinse is ordered to cleanse a deep sore that is not healing. It is then followed by a gentler rinse of warm tap water. The effect lasts about 4 hours, so it should not be used more frequently than instructed. Do not continue using peroxide longer than 7 days. If uncertain about the use of peroxide, talk with the doctor or nurse. Recent research strongly advises against using it.

➤ **Serve soft foods that are easier to swallow.**

Meats and proteins: Include beef, pork, chicken, fish, smooth peanut butter, eggs, cottage cheese, mild cheese, macaroni and cheese, yogurt, and bean casseroles. Always make sure that meat is well cooked, tender, and easy to chew. Avoid sharp cheese, crunchy peanut butter, and spicy foods.

Vegetables: Include well-cooked vegetables that are easy to chew and baked or mashed potatoes. Avoid vegetables with a lot of acid such as tomatoes, potato skins, crunchy or raw vegetables, fried potatoes or vegetables, and tomato soups and sauces.

Fruits: Include applesauce, apple juice, grape juice, nectars, prune juice, soft-cooked or fresh non-citrus fruits, and bananas. Avoid citrus fruits and juices and fruit peels.

Milk: Include milk, milk shakes, cream soups, eggnog, buttermilk, custards, and puddings.

Breads: Include all cooked or dry soft cereals, soft bread and rolls, and pasta with mild sauce. Avoid seeded breads, crusty breads, or granola bars.

➤ **Soften breads and cereals with milk.**

➤ **Use a blender.**

➤ **Use gravy, butter, or cream sauces, which add liquid to food and make it easier to swallow.**

➤ **Eat foods at room temperature.**

➤ **Avoid *extremely* hot or cold foods.**

➤ **Let carbonation or fizz escape from sodas.**

➤ **Serve gelatin, pudding, and softened ice cream.** These foods count as liquids. They are important to offer because the person with mouth sores needs many fluids to combat a dry, sore mouth and throat to prevent dehydration and imbalances of important body chemistry.

➤ **Ask about high-calorie liquids,** such as Ensure™, Isocal™, or milk shake recipes.

➤ **Avoid cigarettes, pipes, chewing tobacco, and alcoholic beverages.**

Prevent mouth sores

If the person does not have mouth sores or ulcers, follow this daily schedule to prevent such problems.

➤ **Brush the teeth at least every 4 hours. Rinse the mouth every 2 hours with salt water or salt water and baking soda. Swish with warm water for at least 1 minute and then spit out the rinse.** Rinsing, even with warm water, removes bacteria and food buildup that can lead to mouth infections and sores. To be effective, the whole mouth care routine should last at least 5 minutes.

➤ **Use any of these to clean the teeth**:

Soft toothbrush

Soft sponge applicator

Cotton-tipped applicator

Finger wrapped with gauze or soft washcloth

The mouth is easily irritated. Softer toothbrushes prevent cutting or scraping and reduce the likelihood of infection.

➤ **Keep lips moist with petroleum jelly, mild lip balm, or cocoa butter.** If swallowing is difficult, then the mouth and lips become dry. Lip balms prevent chapping and infection.

➤ **Drink about 2 to 3 quarts of fluid each day**—unless otherwise ordered.

➤ **Chew sugarless gum or use sugarless hard candies,** which moisten the mouth. They increase saliva in the mouth. Sugarless products are recommended because they limit the buildup of bacteria. Taking frequent sips of water also helps. Many people carry large plastic cups with straws attached and drink from these frequently to keep the mouth moist.

➤ **Set a Water-Pik™ on the *lowest* setting, if one is used.** Water from a Water-Pik™ can cause bleeding. The gums are very sensitive as a side effect of some chemotherapy drugs, and they bleed easily.

➤ **Use dental floss at bedtime.** Flossing removes food particles but can also cause small cuts. These heal during the night because no food is eaten for at least 8 or 10 hours. However, flossing should be avoided when platelet or white blood cell counts are low to prevent infection and bleeding. <u>Do not floss if it causes bleeding or pain</u>.

➤ **Remove dentures when rinsing or sleeping.** Dentures irritate a dry mouth. They can cause enough scraping to break the skin and start an infection, especially if they don't fit well.

➤ **Avoid commercial mouthwashes.** Many commercial mouthwashes have alcohol in them, which is drying. Ask the nurses what works best and what mouthwashes are recommended.

➤ **Avoid glycerine or lemon juice mouth swabs.** They are also drying. Avoid using them because the skin inside the mouth can crack and get infected when it's dry.

Possible Obstacles

Here are some obstacles that have sometimes stopped others from carrying out their plans to solve mouth sore problems

1. "He doesn't want to quit smoking or drinking."

   Response: Both of these habits irritate the mouth. <u>If the person on chemotherapy doesn't quit either habit, then that's all the more reason to do other things to take care of the mouth, such as frequent rinsing</u>.

2. "It's upsetting for him to have soft or mashed foods."

   Response: <u>Serve soft foods attractively. Add flavorings that the person likes. Encourage everyone in the family to eat the same or similar foods</u>.

Think of *other* obstacles that could interfere with carrying out your plan

What additional road blocks could get in the way of doing the things recommended in this home care plan? For example, will the person with cancer cooperate? Will other people help? How will you explain your needs to other people? Do you have the time and energy to carry out the plan?

You need to develop plans for getting around these road blocks. Use the four COPE ideas (creativity, optimism, planning, and expert information) in developing your plans. See the chapter on Solving Home Care Problems at the beginning of the book for a discussion of how to use the four COPE ideas in overcoming your obstacles.

Carrying Out and Adjusting Your Plan

Carrying out your plan

The most important thing you can do is to set up and follow a regular, daily schedule for treating and preventing mouth sores.

Checking on results

Check regularly with the person with cancer on how troublesome and uncomfortable the mouth sores are. Pay special attention to whether they interfere with eating.

Sore Mouth

If your plan doesn't work

If problems with mouth soreness or swallowing are getting worse, review this home care plan and ask yourself if you are doing everything you can to encourage good oral hygiene and to protect the mouth and throat against soreness and infection. <u>Tell the doctor or nurse what was done to deal with the mouth problems and discuss what else they think should be done</u>.

Nausea and Vomiting

Overview of the
Home Care Plan for Nausea and Vomiting

Understanding the Problem

There has been great progess in the past few years in controlling nausea with cancer treatments

Different people have different amounts of nausea, depending on their treatments and their reactions to the treatments

When To Get Professional Help

Symptoms that require professional help

Facts to know when you call for help

What to say when you call

What You Can Do To Help

Make the best use of nausea medicine

What you can do on your own to limit nausea and vomiting

Possible Obstacles

"The person with cancer must take other medicines which make him nauseated."

Carrying Out and Adjusting Your Plan

Keep track of frequency and severity of vomiting and how much nausea interferes with daily activities

If problems persist, ask for other antinausea medicines

(Topics with an arrow in front of them are actions you can take or symptoms you can look for.)

Nausea and Vomiting

[The information in this home care plan fits most situations, but yours may be different.

If the doctor or nurse tells you to do something else, follow what they say. If you think there may be a medical emergency, see pages 65–66.]

Understanding the Problem

It's natural to be concerned about nausea and vomiting. In the last few years, we have learned a great deal about how to control both. As a result, most people receiving treatments for cancer have much less nausea.

Some people never experience any nausea or vomiting from cancer, its treatments, or other medicines. Other people deal with one or both symptoms at different times in their illness, depending on which treatments they receive and how they react to them.

Sometimes, after several treatments, which have made a person nauseated, he or she may feel nausea when seeing or smelling something associated with the treatments. For example, the smell of the treatment room or the sight of the nurse or doctor who gave the treatments may cause nausea and even vomiting. This is a normal reaction. It is due to "conditioning" and will usually go away after treatments are over, when the sights or smells become linked to experiences other than nausea.

Your goals are to:

call for help if it is needed,

make the best use of antinausea medicines, and

do what you can to ease the nausea and vomiting.

When To Get Professional Help

You should have the doctor and nurse fill in the blanks below. Call them if any of the following conditions exist:

➤ **There is blood or "coffee ground" looking material in the vomit.** Coffee ground material is really old blood and signals that some bleeding has occurred inside. This happens rarely, but it is important to report.

➤ **There is vomiting more than ___ times an hour for more than ___ hours.** Ask the doctor or nurse about these times. For most people, vomiting three times per hour for more than 12 hours is serious, but your situation may be different.

➤ **The vomit shoots out for a distance (projectile vomiting).** Projectile vomiting may mean that there are problems in the stomach or intestine that should be investigated by your doctor.

➤ **Two doses of any prescribed medicines are not taken or kept down because of nausea or vomiting.** Medicines will have to be given other ways until pills can stay down again.

➤ **Less than ___ cups of liquid are taken in 24 hours and no solid food is eaten.** <u>Ask the doctor or nurse about the number of cups of liquid</u>. Without liquids, people become dehydrated after continued vomiting. Food is needed to keep up one's energy and to fight the illness. Most people need to drink more than 4 cups in 24 hours. Also, for most people, 2 days without food is dangerous. But your needs may be different, so ask the doctor or nurse when to call about not eating or drinking.

➤ **Weakness or dizziness happens along with the nausea or vomiting.** It is normal to feel a little weak or dizzy with nausea, but if a person can't get up, then you need to call a doctor or nurse.

➤ **Severe stomach pain happens while vomiting.** <u>Severe pain is always a reason to call the doctor.</u>

When you call, you will need to know the following facts to answer questions that the doctor or nurse may ask you

1. How long has nausea been a problem?

2. When does it begin and how long does it last?

3. How bad was the most recent nausea?

4. How much does the nausea interfere with normal activities?

5. Was medicine prescribed for nausea or vomiting?

   Name of medicine(s)
   How often should it be taken?
   How many pills at one time?
   How many pills were taken in the last 2 days?
   How much relief did it give?
   How long did the relief last?

6. In addition to giving medicine for nausea, what was done to help the person with nausea to feel better and what were the results?

7. Was the nausea followed by vomiting?

8. What did the vomit look like? Was this vomit the same color as earlier vomit? If not, how was it different?

9. How often has vomiting happened in the last 24 hours?

10. What other symptoms are new since the nausea or vomiting began? (Answer questions below for each new symptom.)

    SYMPTOM: _____

    Where is it? _____

    How bad is it? _____

    When did it start? _____

    When does it happen? _____

    How long does it last? _____

    What relieves it? _____

    What doesn't help?_____

11. What and how much was eaten in the last 24 hours?

12. What and how much liquid was taken in the last 24 hours?

13. How frequent were bowel movements in the last 2 days, and were they the same amount and color as usual?

14. What is the temperature of the person with nausea?

15. When was the last cancer treatment?

Here is an example of what you might say when calling

"I am Joan Smith, Harry Smith's wife. My husband is Dr. Harvey's patient. The home care plan for nausea says that I should call if he vomited after taking the last two doses of his antinausea medicine. I'm worried that his nausea is a lot worse now."

What You Can Do To Help

There are two things you can do at home to deal with a nausea or vomiting problem:

make the best use of nausea medicine, and

what you can do to limit nausea and vomiting.

Make the best use of nausea medicine

Check to be sure you followed the instructions on the label and the instructions given by the nursing staff. Here are ways to get the most help from antinausea medicine, especially around the time of chemotherapy treatments.

➤ **Take antinausea medicine on a consistent schedule.** Take the prescribed antinausea medicine before chemotherapy treatment. Continue to take the medicine every 4 to 6 hours or as prescribed for at least 12 to 24 hours, and continue as long as nausea or vomiting persists. The antinausea medicine must be taken on a consistent schedule to maintain enough of the drug in the blood.

➤ **Take antinausea medicine before and after receiving chemotherapy treatments.** Take pills with chemotherapy. For the medicine to be effective, you need to have enough in your blood. That's why it should be taken before chemotherapy and then continued every 4 to 6 hours or as directed by the doctor.

A sample schedule of medicine might look like this:

At bedtime before treatments

The morning before treatments

4 to 6 hours after treatments

➤ **Take antinausea medicines one-half hour before meals.** The antinausea medicine helps the person with cancer get ready to eat and have an appetite.

What you can do to limit nausea and vomiting

This is a list of ideas for what you can do to help reduce nausea and vomiting. Start with those ideas that have helped in the past, but try new ideas, too. You can't be sure if an idea will help until you try.

➤ **Encourage eating 3 to 4 hours before treatment but not just before treatment.** Eat frequent light meals during the day. This keeps something in the stomach and helps the body to get the nutrition it needs. Try to have the stomach empty just before treatments if you find that works best for you.

➤ **Avoid serving fried foods, dairy products, and acids such as fruit juices or vinegar salad dressings.** Fried and acidic foods are hard to digest and may make nausea worse.

➤ **Offer chewing gum or hard candy.** Try peppermint or fruit flavors. They cover up unpleasant tastes during chemotherapy.

➤ **Let fresh air into the house or have the person go outside.** Taking in more oxygen helps calm the stomach and can decrease feelings of nausea. Encourage mouth breathing for a few minutes or open a window.

➤ **Encourage rest.** Some people find it helpful to lie down when they are nauseated. The antinausea medicine often makes people sleepy and helps them to rest through their nausea.

Allow short rest times between everyday activities such as dressing or walking. Taking it easy can help to keep the nausea away.

➤ **Offer sips of fluid 2 hours after vomiting.** Wait awhile before offering food or drink. Then offer 1 or 2 ounces of fluid at a time. Let the fizz go out of sodas before drinking them because carbonation can upset the stomach again. Stir sodas vigorously with a spoon to release carbonation, leave the can open, or leave the cap off.

➤ **Offer dry crackers.** This often helps women who are pregnant and nauseated. Crackers help many people with cancer, too.

➤ **Avoid unpleasant or strong odors.** It may help the person with cancer to stay away from the kitchen. If odors are in the kitchen, breathe through the mouth and not through the nose, if possible.

➤ **Encourage frequent mouth rinses.** Frequent swishing and rinsing remove unpleasant tastes that can upset the stomach.

➤ **Suggest wearing loosely fitting clothes.** Avoid tight-fitting material, especially around the waist or neck. These put pressure on the throat and stomach and add to stomach upset.

➤ **Distract their attention.** Watching television or reading may help to distract the person with nausea.

➤ **Encourage relaxing.** If the person with cancer is tense, physical symptoms also seem more intense. Many people find that by relaxing, the symptoms are not as bothersome. (See the home care plan for Coping with Anxiety for a detailed explanation of how to practice relaxation.)

➤ **Take another person to treatments.** A companion can show support and can help the person with cancer think and talk about other things besides the nausea and treatment.

Possible Obstacles

Here is an obstacle that other people have faced when treating nausea

1. "Some other medicines that he takes make him sick to the stomach and he *can't* stop taking those other pills. They make him sick as soon as they are swallowed, and I don't know what to do about that."

   Response: <u>If the person with cancer must take other pills, then never give them on an empty stomach unless the label</u>

instructs you to do so. Otherwise, offer Maalox™, dry bread, or saltines beforehand, or give the medicine after a meal.

If the person with nausea is taking potassium pills or potassium liquid, talk with the pharmacist or nurse about its side effects. A common one is nausea, which can make the nausea from chemotherapy worse. You can often get the form of the potassium medicine changed by talking over the nausea problem with the doctor. A new form of potassium pill may reduce the nausea.

Think of *other* obstacles that could interfere with carrying out your plan

What additional road blocks could get in the way of doing the things recommended in this home care plan? For example, will the person with cancer cooperate? Will other people help? How will you explain your needs to other people? Do you have the time and energy to carry out the plan?

You need to develop plans for getting around these road blocks. Use the four COPE ideas (creativity, optimism, planning, and expert information) in developing your plans. See the chapter on Solving Home Care Problems at the beginning of the book for a discussion of how to use the four COPE ideas in overcoming your obstacles.

Carrying Out and Adjusting Your Plan

Checking on results

You can check on how well this home care plan is working by keeping track of the number of times the person with cancer vomited, by asking how severe the feelings of nausea are, and by noticing how much he or she has cut back on normal activities because of nausea.

If your plan doesn't work

If problems with nausea are getting worse, review the list under When To Get Professional Help in this plan. Ask yourself if you are doing everything you can to reduce this symptom. If the person is becoming anxious about getting nauseated or if the nausea is harder and harder to control, ask the doctor about other antinausea medicines or about reducing the chemotherapy dose.

Diarrhea

Overview of the
Home Care Plan for Diarrhea

Understanding the Problem

What is diarrhea?

Why is it important to control diarrhea?

When To Get Professional Help

Situations and symptoms that require professional help

Facts to know when you call for help

What to say

What You Can Do To Help

Give medicines for diarrhea

Replace lost fluids and nutrients

Avoid certain foods

Increase comfort

Possible Obstacles

"He's had nothing to eat for days, so this diarrhea can't last much longer."

Carrying Out and Adjusting Your Plan

Keep track of frequency and severity of diarrhea

Report unresolved problems to medical staff

(Topics with an arrow in front of them are actions you can take or symptoms you can look for.)

Diarrhea

[The information in this home care plan fits most situations, but yours may be different.

If the doctor or nurse tells you to do something else, follow what they say. If you think there may be a medical emergency, see pages 73–74.]

Understanding the Problem

Diarrhea is defined as liquid stools. With diarrhea, bowel movements can happen more frequently and feel more urgent. Having diarrhea can also be very upsetting. It is caused by cancer treatments, cancer medicines, and other medicines, and sometimes emotional distress. Losing these fluids adds to fatigue and feeling "washed out." Diarrhea can also cause dehydration, which can be a serious health problem. Therefore, stopping diarrhea is important for comfort and health.

Your goals are to:

call for professional help when it is needed,

be sure diarrhea medicines are taken,

replace lost fluids and nutrients after vomiting,

help the person with cancer avoid certain foods, and

do what you can to increase comfort.

When To Get Professional Help

All of these "call now" problems demand quick attention because there is a danger that too much fluid is being lost. Serious health problems can result if a person is dehydrated for a long time.

Call the doctor or nurse if any of the following conditions exist

➤ **Severe diarrhea.** Ask the doctor or nurse when to call about diarrhea. Severe diarrhea means that a lot of fluid is being lost. With severe diarrhea, stools are very runny, and the person often complains of stomach cramps as well. The severity of the problem depends on many factors, such as the person's weight or previous state of fluid balance.

Diarrhea

Losing small amounts of fluid and stool in diarrhea can be dangerous for a small, thin person or for anyone who has recently been struggling with diarrhea or vomiting. In this situation, dehydration happens quickly. Reporting severe diarrhea early is important so that medicines and fluids can be given to stop the diarrhea and to reverse or correct the dehydration.

➤ **Diarrhea for more than 1 day.**

➤ **Blood in the diarrhea stool.**

➤ **Fever above 100.4 °F with diarrhea.**

Know the following facts before you call

1. How many bowel movements are usual each day?

2. How many bowel movements have there been in the last 24 hours?

3. How runny were they?

4. Are there any other symptoms with the diarrhea?

   ___ stomach pain

   ___ stomach cramps

   ___ bloating (feeling very full in the stomach or abdomen)

   ___ nausea (sick to the stomach)

   ___ vomiting

   ___ fever

   ___ blood in the diarrhea

   Information about other symptoms helps the doctor or nurse to know how serious the problem is. Other side effects can be a danger, such as a rectal infection or dehydration. Rectal infections are caused by bacteria that invade the body when the skin is broken from the acids and irritants in the diarrhea stool. This is uncomfortable and painful.

5. How much liquid was taken and how much was eaten in the last 2 days?

   Knowing the approximate amounts of liquids and foods taken helps the doctor and nurse to know if the body is receiving enough to replace what is being lost. Dehydration is important to treat because it could lead to dangerously low blood pressure and chemical imbalance in the body. Sometimes intravenous (IV) fluids are ordered to balance the fluid loss and put important fluids, water, vitamins, and minerals back into the body. For example, IV fluids can contain other nutrients that are being lost in the diarrhea, such as glucose, potassium, and sodium.

6. What medicines were taken in the last 2 to 3 days?

   ___ chemotherapy (when?)

   ___ laxatives

   ___ antidiarrhea tablets or liquids

7. Has weight been lost? How much?

8. Is there any history of other bowel problems, such as diverticulitis, colitis, or irritable bowel syndrome?

Here is an example of what you might say when calling for help

"I am Joan Smith, Harry Smith's wife. My husband is a patient of Dr. Harvey's. The home care plan on diarrhea says to call if he's had diarrhea for more than one day. He has, and he's getting pretty weak."

What You Can Do To Help

There are four things you can do to solve this problem. Consider them in this order:

give medicines for diarrhea,

replace lost fluids and nutrients,

avoid certain foods, and

increase comfort.

Give medicines for diarrhea

Antidiarrhea medicine is a fast way to stop this problem. These medicines slow down the bowel.

➤ **Check with the doctor or nurse before you give diarrhea medicines that you can buy without a prescription.** The doctor might prefer that you use a prescription medicine or certain "over-the-counter" drugs to stop diarrhea, or he or she may decide that a prescription is not needed.

➤ **Follow the instructions on the bottle or on the prescription.** Sometimes antidiarrheal medicines do the job too well. If too much is given, they can cause cramping and constipation. The person may get very sleepy if given too much because these medicines cause sleepiness.

Replace lost fluids and nutrients

Important fluids are lost with diarrheal stool. Replacing them is crucial. Here are several ways to do this:

➤ **Offer clear liquids,** for example, chicken broth; tea; apple, cranberry, or grape juice; ginger ale; Popsicles™; and Gatorade™. They provide important food but also let the bowel rest. Clear liquids are easier for the intestines to absorb into the bloodstream, and they begin to replace the fluids being lost with diarrhea.

➤ **Serve fluids between meals.** Taking fluids between meals keeps a steady amount of water and other nutrients entering the body. Drinking between meals is less likely to cramp a sore stomach or intestines.

➤ **Serve low-fiber foods,** for example, bananas, rice, applesauce, mashed potatoes, dry toast, crackers, eggs, fish, poultry, cottage cheese, and yogurt. Low-fiber foods do not attract or pull water out of the body into the bowel. They are easier to digest than high-fiber vegetables.

➤ **Eat small meals throughout the day instead of three larger meals.** Smaller meals are easier to digest. The person takes in more fluid and food if meals are served more often than three times a day.

➤ **Increase high-potassium foods in the diet,** such as apricot or peach nectar, bananas, and mashed or baked potatoes. People tend to lose potassium when they have diarrhea. This chemical is vital to the body and needs to be replaced.

Avoid certain foods

Some foods increase the action of the bowel and how quickly it pulls fluid out of body tissues into stool. Avoiding these foods helps to reduce problems with diarrhea.

➤ **Avoid serving foods that produce gas,** for example, beans, raw vegetables, raw fruits, broccoli, corn, cabbage, cauliflower, carbonated drinks, and chewing gum. These foods cause a feeling of fullness and makes a person stop eating or drinking earlier. Gas also adds to discomfort. Chewing gum should also be avoided because it makes some people swallow air, which also adds to abdominal discomfort.

➤ **Avoid serving foods that contain acids,** such as highly spiced food or citrus juices like orange or grapefruit. These make the stomach and intestines churn and can create more discomfort as well as more diarrhea.

➤ **Avoid serving fat,** such as fatty meats and greasy fried foods. Fats are difficult to digest. If the person has diarrhea, then fats are pushed through the intestines without being digested. Undigested fat increases problems with diarrhea.

➤ **Cool down hot food or hot drinks.** Hot foods and liquids make the bowels move. Avoid these until the problem with diarrhea is solved.

➤ **Limit caffeine intake,** for example, coffee, strong teas, sodas with caffeine, and chocolate. Caffeine makes the bowel work faster. If a person has diarrhea, you want to slow down his or her bowels, which are already overactive.

➤ **Avoid giving milk and milk products if they seem to make diarrhea worse.** Milk can make diarrhea worse. It can also cause stomach cramps in some adults.

Increase comfort

The lower abdomen can become quite sore from intestinal cramps that may accompany diarrhea. The person with cancer can also feel worn out from bouts with diarrhea. Rectal skin or skin around a stoma (an opening in the skin on the abdomen for stool to come out into a bag) can become very sore. Here are several ways to ease abdominal or skin soreness:

➤ **Put a warm water bottle wrapped in a towel on the abdomen.** Warmth on the stomach can relieve pain and discomfort caused by stomach tightness or cramps. However, do not use a heating pad or very hot water in the water bottle. The skin may be sensitive to heat, especially if the person is receiving chemotherapy or radiation therapy, and a heating pad or very hot water bottle could cause problems with the skin.

➤ **Cleanse rectal area.** After diarrhea, cleanse the outside of the rectum gently with warm water and then dry the skin to reduce redness and prevent infection.

➤ **Soak in warm water.** Use a tub or Sitz™ bath. Sitz™ baths can be bought at most pharmacies or medical equipment stores. Sitz™ baths are plastic bowls that are placed over the toilet; the person can sit in the bowl of warm water while it flows into the bowl from above and spills into the toilet below. Sitting in a tub of warm water is also practical.

➤ **Apply soothing creams, ointments, or astringent pads such as Tucks™ to the rectal area.** Creams prevent rectal skin from chapping in the same way that they prevent diaper rash or chapping on infants' skin. Try Nupercainal™, A&D™, or Vaseline™. Astringent pads also help to dry the area and soothe irritated skin.

Protect the rectal skin with an ointment such as Desitin™. If diarrhea continues and the rectal area becomes very sore and red, apply an ointment such as Desitin™ to cover the skin. Fluids will be less likely to burn the skin since this type of ointment covers the skin with a protective layer.

If the person with cancer has a stoma and the skin around the opening becomes irritated, talk to an enterostomal therapy nurse for recommendations.

Possible Obstacles

Think about what ideas or attitudes might prevent you from carrying out your plan and reaching the goal of controlling or preventing diarrhea.

Here is one obstacle that other people have faced

1. "He's had nothing to eat or drink for days, so this diarrhea can't last much longer."

    Response: The body can keep removing fluid for much longer than you think. The fluid is drawn from body tissues, and diarrhea can continue even if the person stops eating or drinking for days. It's important to replace the fluids that are lost even if the person thinks that these will be washed out instantly.

Think of *other* obstacles that could interfere with carrying out your plan

What additional road blocks could get in the way of doing the things recommended in this home care plan? For example, will the person with cancer cooperate? Will other people help? How will you explain your needs to other people? Do you have the time and energy to carry out the plan?

You need to develop plans for getting around these road blocks. Use the four COPE ideas (creativity, optimism, planning, and expert information) in developing your plans. See the chapter on Solving Home Care Problems at the beginning of the book for a discussion of how to use the four COPE ideas in overcoming your obstacles.

Carrying Out and Adjusting Your Plan

Checking on results

Be aware of the frequency and severity of diarrhea. Are you able to stop the diarrhea on your own whenever it starts? Is the rectal skin or skin around a stoma as well cared for and protected as it can be? Are other precautions with fluids and diet being followed to prevent diarrhea?

If your plan doesn't work

If problems with diarrhea are getting worse or the person with cancer is becoming worn out, review the section on When To Get Professional Help in this plan. When calling, tell the doctor or nurse what was done to deal with diarrhea and discuss what else should be done.

If diarrhea isn't severe but continues for several days, ask the doctor or nurse for help. Tell them what you have done and what the results have been.

Diarrhea

Constipation

Overview of the
Home Care Plan for Constipation

Understanding the Problem

What constipation is

What causes constipation

Why it is important to control constipation

When To Get Professional Help

Symptoms that require professional help

Facts to know when you call

What to say

What You Can Do To Help

Relieve constipation

Prevent constipation

Possible Obstacles

"She hasn't eaten, so how could she be constipated?"

"He's embarrassed to talk about his constipation to me."

Carrying Out and Adjusting Your Plan

Plan in advance to prevent constipation

Keep track of bowel habits

Report continued problems to medical staff

(Topics with an arrow in front of them are actions you can take or symptoms you can look for.)

Constipation

[The information in this home care plan fits most situations, but yours may be different.

If the doctor or nurse tells you to do something else, follow what they say. If you think there may be a medical emergency, see pages 83–84.]

Understanding the Problem

Constipation occurs when bowel movements happen less often than usual and when stools are hard or difficult to move. Constipation can be caused by medicines used to treat cancer, narcotics, emotional stress, changes in diet, or decreases in activity. Even if the person with cancer isn't eating much, the body still makes waste, and regular bowel movements are necessary. Constipation can also be very uncomfortable.

When persons with cancer are constipated, they often have a decreased appetite and feel bloated. These feelings add to their discomfort.

Your goals are to:

call for professional help when it is needed,

help to relieve the constipation, and

prevent it in the future.

When To Get Professional Help

Call the doctor or nurse if any of the following conditions exist

➤ **The normal routine was once a day and he or she has not had a bowel movement in 3 or 4 days** OR

The normal routine was once every other day and he or she has not had a bowel movement in 4 or 5 days. The person with cancer becomes more uncomfortable as the constipation continues. If it is allowed to continue for more than a few days, it will also be more difficult to reverse. Reporting the usual bowel pattern and the day and type of the last movement helps the doctor or nurse to suggest medications and to advise you on other measures to take to help relieve the problem. If the doctor or nurse knows that there are smears of stool on the clothes or the person with cancer feels full in the rectal area, then they know that the lower bowel needs to be evacuated. A laxative or stool softener needs to be prescribed to help with the emptying of the lower bowel in the future.

➤ **Severe straining on the toilet or commode** OR

Severe abdominal pain or an abdomen that feels harder than normal and very full OR

Red blood around the outside of the stools or problems with hemorrhoids. Reporting other symptoms alerts the health professionals to assess whether or not other more serious problems are happening. In these situations, constipation is a sign or side effect of further problems. Pain or vomiting can indicate an abdominal problem, such as a temporary blocking of a section of the bowel. A tumor may also be pressing on a part of the bowel and preventing that part from allowing stool to pass through it in a normal pattern. Report any pain or bleeding.

When you call you will need to know the answers to the following questions

The doctor or nurse may ask you these questions, which assess whether or not the constipation is increasing in severity and whether or not there is stool close to the rectum but the muscles are not moving the stool out.

1. How often are the person's usual bowel movements?

2. When was the last bowel movement? What did it look like?

   Reporting what the last bowel movement looked like (watery or dry) tells the health professional if food is being digested properly and if the stool has enough water in it as it passes through the long digestive and intestinal tract. In addition, color is important to report. Very dark stools could indicate blood in the stool unless the person normally takes iron, which turns the stool darker.

3. Does the person normally take medicines to help move the bowels, such as laxatives, stool softeners, Metamucil™, Citrucel™, or suppositories?

4. Does feeling constipated interfere with normal activities, such as walking or eating?

   The degree to which the constipation is interfering with the person's comfort and activities is important to report because it helps the health professional decide what actions should be taken to relieve the constipation.

5. What other symptoms are there?

___ distention or bloating of the abdomen

___ a pressure or sense of fullness in the rectal area

___ small, frequent "smears" of stool

___ small amounts of loose stools or "leaking"

___ rectal pain with a bowel movement

___ constantly feeling the need to have a bowel movement but unable to pass stool

___ small amounts of loose stool or diarrhea

Answers to questions about other symptoms related to the lower bowel help the doctor or nurse understand what might be stopping final evacuation. If there is no bowel movement for days, but small amounts of diarrhea occur, they may recommend a gentle enema or a visit to the clinic for a rectal exam and further assessment.

6. What medications were taken in the last 2 to 3 days?

___ narcotics

___ laxatives

___ chemotherapy

Some medicines can interrupt normal bowel activity, and the doctor or nurse will recognize which pills might be contributing to constipation. Be sure to mention any medicines that are being taken.

7. What and how much was eaten or drunk in the last 24 hours?

If health professionals know about food and fluid intake, they can judge if the constipation may cause an emergency requiring a clinic visit. If they decide that the relief of constipation is not an emergency, they may suggest an increase in fluids as well as many of the actions that are listed on the following pages.

Here is an example of what you might say when calling

"I am Joan Smith, Harry Smith's wife. My husband is Dr. Harvey's patient. The home care plan for constipation says to call if he hasn't had a bowel movement for 4 days. He feels like he should go, but nothing happens."

What You Can Do To Help

There are two things you can do to help solve a constipation problem:

relieve constipation, and

prevent it in the future.

Relieve constipation

➤ **Give oral laxatives that have stool softeners in them and use them every day.** Start with two at night. Add two after breakfast if there is no relief. Continue taking two to four laxative tablets every day.

Laxatives relieve constipation by stimulating the bowels to move waste products out of the body. Stool softeners draw water into the bowel and decrease the dryness of stools so that stool moves down the long intestinal tract more easily. The combination of both laxatives and stool softeners gives the best results. Tablets can be bought at any pharmacy. There are many brands to choose from, but Senokot-S™ tablets are frequently recommended by cancer pain specialists. If finances are a concern, ask the pharmacist about less expensive medicines, or ask the doctor or nurse if they have office samples.

➤ **Increase the number of tablets.** Take three laxative tablets with stool softeners at night if the previous laxative schedule fails. Different people require different amounts of these medicines. You can increase the number of tablets up to eight a day. People taking pain medicine may need as many as six to eight a day to prevent constipation from the pain medicine. Report side effects that are warned about on the label to a doctor or nurse (for example, severe stomach cramping, nausea, or vomiting).

OR

Take three laxative tablets at bedtime *and* after breakfast if there is still no relief.

➤ **Give a rectal suppository.** Suppositories can be inserted in the rectum, where they stimulate the lower bowel to move. Many people store suppositories in the refrigerator. However, suppositories should not be used if the person with cancer has low platelet or white blood cell counts; there is a risk of infection or bleeding if the suppository breaks a small blood vessel in the rectal area.

➤ **Give enemas after checking with the doctor or nurse.** Give a mineral oil enema, Fleets™ enema, or soap suds enema for immediate relief, but first check with the health care staff. Enemas are the last step to try for relieving constipation. They evacuate the lower bowel, which helps the upper bowel move as well. There are three basic kinds of enemas. An oil enema softens stool. Usually, a small amount of mineral oil (4 ounces) is pushed gently into the bowel through a small plastic bottle. Then the person holds the oil in until feeling the urge to have a bowel movement. A Fleets™ enema puts about 4 ounces of chemically treated (sodium phosphate or sodium biphosphate) water into the bowel along with medicines such as castor oil or laxatives. A soap suds enema is made at home. Mix four to eight ounces of warm water with a small amount of dish soap, and then place this in a plastic enema bag. The end of the bag is lubricated with oil or vaseline and inserted into the rectum. Then, the suds mixture is dripped slowly into the lower bowel. The bowels move because the sheer volume of the liquid stimulates movement and because the soap suds mildly irritate the bowel. All of these enemas and equipment can be bought at a pharmacy. A new, very small, easy-to-use enema (two inches long) has just been marketed. It is easy to insert and works well.

Only 1 or 2 enemas should be needed to relieve constipation. It is best to give an enema with the person lying on his or her left side near a bathroom or with a commode next to the bed or couch.

Prevent constipation

There are many things you can do to prevent constipation. If the person with cancer has been constipated recently, then you should use these strategies to prevent it.

➤ **Gradually add foods high in fiber to the diet,** such as

> whole grain cereals and breads,
>
> dried fruits such as prunes and raisins,
>
> popcorn, nuts, and seeds,
>
> beans and legumes, and
>
> raw fruits and vegetables.

High-fiber foods draw water into the stools. They also provide bulk—that is, they are made of materials that do not break down as the food passes through the intestines, where it is normally dissolved by acids and enzymes. For example, skins and coverings on nuts, beans, grains, fruits, and vegetables are not easily broken down, and these help form stools that are easily passed out of the body. If raw fruits and vegetables are hard to chew, try grating or cooking them.

➤ **Add unprocessed bran to the diet.** Bran stimulates bowel activity. Sprinkle it on cereal. Start with 2 teaspoons per day and gradually increase this amount up to 2 tablespoons per day. Be careful. Adding large amounts of bran too quickly to the diet might cause diarrhea and discomfort.

➤ **Encourage the drinking of plenty of fluids,** up to 6 to 8 glasses of liquid every day. Fluids add water to the stools and prevent constipation caused by dry, hard stools.

➤ **Offer hot or warm liquids.** They stimulate the bowels. People often say that coffee makes them go to the bathroom. It's the combination of caffeine and hot liquid that causes this.

➤ **Serve prune juice, hot lemon water, or tea.** Prune juice, whether warm or cold, and hot lemon water or tea all stimulate the bowels.

➤ **Exercise, such as walking every day, helps.** Even a small amount of movement, such as walking in the house, helps stimulate muscles that make the bowel work. Talk to the doctor about the amount and type of exercise that is best for the person with cancer.

➤ **Avoid regular use of enemas, if possible.** Enemas may prevent the intestines from finding a regular pattern.

➤ **Give one or two stool softeners every day, and use a laxative if taking narcotics.** One or two stool softeners every day help to prevent constipation. If the person is eating or drinking less and not feeling well enough to exercise, then stool softeners should be tried. Narcotics also cause constipation, so give a daily laxative and read the home care plan on Cancer Pain for a more complete explanation of using laxatives with narcotics.

➤ **Maintain a daily schedule of prevention.** First, try diet and exercise, then medicines, and follow a daily schedule just the way you do with other medicines. Following a schedule of diet, exercise, and medicines to prevent constipation should be considered as important as taking other medicines. Daily attention to eating helpful foods, drinking liquids, and taking preventive medicines will add up to successful prevention.

Possible Obstacles

Constipation is a common problem for people who are weak, spend a lot of time in bed, and are not eating.

Here are some obstacles that others have faced in solving this problem

1. "She hasn't eaten much all month. How could anything be in there to plug her up or make her constipated?"

   Response: <u>The body makes waste products and stool even when people eat very little</u>. Taking narcotics or not walking much also makes constipation more likely to happen. Laxatives and sometimes enemas are needed to get the bowels moving.

2. "He's too embarrassed about his constipation to tell me about it—so how can I help him?"

   Response: <u>Put him in charge of his own care</u>. Have him read this home care plan. It possible, he should understand what causes constipation and what to do about it. Then he can be responsible for managing it. Another strategy is to have him talk directly to a nurse. Most people are willing to talk about "embarrassing" things to health professionals. Also, health professionals are experienced in discussing these subjects without embarrassment.

Think of *other* obstacles that could interfere with carrying out your plan

What additional road blocks could get in the way of doing the things recommended in this home care plan? For example, will the person with cancer cooperate? Will other people help? How will you explain your needs to other people? Do you have the time and energy to carry out the plan?

You need to develop plans for getting around these road blocks. Use the four COPE ideas (creativity, optimism, planning, and expert information) in developing your plans. See the chapter on Solving Home Care Problems at the beginning of the book for a discussion of how to use the four COPE ideas in overcoming your obstacles.

Carrying Out and Adjusting Your Plan

Carrying out your plan

<u>Prepare in advance for constipation, especially if narcotics are prescribed or if the person is less active</u>. Use this home care plan as a reference and begin to change diet and food habits to prevent constipation.

Checking on results

<u>After new medicines are started, ask the person with cancer if bowel habits are changing</u>. Is the constipation happening less frequently? When it does happen, do you both know what to do to relieve it? Are actions to prevent constipation taking effect?

If your plan doesn't work

If your plan does not seem to be working or constipation is getting worse, there are three things you can do. Consider them in this order.

1. Check the When To Get Professional Help section of this care plan. If you answer "yes" to any of those questions, call the doctor or nurse immediately.

2. Review the strategies in the section on What You Can Do To Help in this care plan to be sure you are doing everything you can to deal with this problem.

3. <u>If constipation continues, ask the doctor or nurse for help</u>. Tell them what you have done and what the results have been.

Cancer Pain

Overview of the
Home Care Plan for Cancer Pain

Understanding the Problem

Cancer pain can be controlled

The person with cancer has a right to good pain control

Part of your job is to be sure of good pain control

Pain control takes time to achieve, so persist

Only the person with pain knows what the pain is like

Don't assume that pain means that cancer is spreading

How doctors use the "pain ladder" to control pain

When To Get Professional Help

Symptoms that require immediate professional help for pain

Facts you need and what to say when you call

Symptoms that require immediate professional help for the effects of pain medicines

Facts you need when you call about effects of pain medicines

When to call for help during regular office hours

What You Can Do To Help

Make the best use of medicines

Understand the medication plan

Ask about changing pain prescriptions

Manage common side effects of pain medicine

Prevent and control pain on your own

Possible Obstacles

"I'm afraid of addiction."

"I want to 'save' the pain medicine until the pain is severe."

"No one wants to hear about my pain."

"Only people who are dying take morphine."

Carrying Out and Adjusting Your Plan

Keep track of pain levels

Be sure that the person with pain understands and fully accepts the pain ratings

Do not accept anything less than the best pain control

If necessary, ask for referral to a cancer pain specialist

(Topics with an arrow in front of them are actions you can take or symptoms you can look for.)

Cancer Pain

[The information in this home care plan fits most situations, but yours may be different.

If the doctor or nurse tells you to do something else, follow what they say. If you think there may be a medical emergency, see pages 96–97.]

Understanding the Problem

Most cancer pain can be eliminated, and all cancer pain can be controlled.

Every person with cancer has the right to good pain control. Your job, as a home caregiver, is to be sure that happens.

It takes time to get good pain control, so be patient. On the other hand, do not give up until adequate pain control is achieved.

When many people think of cancer, they think of pain. But today, most cancer pain can be eliminated. For example, even in cases of advanced cancer, pain has been controlled in 90% to 99% of those persons who are helped by hospice workers. In 9 out of 10 cases, physicians can control cancer pain by using pills alone. They do not have to use injections, operations, or other pain control methods. In these few situations in which pain cannot be totally eliminated, it can be reduced so that the person with cancer can live with it day to day and accomplish activities that are important to him or her.

People with cancer and their home caregivers must tell the doctors and nurses how pain gets in the way of doing normal everyday activities, such as moving around or dressing. This information is useful to doctors in evaluating pain and in developing an effective treatment plan to control it.

It is also important that everyone be open and supportive about controlling pain. Family and friends should make clear that they believe the person's pain reports. People with pain are the only people who know how much pain they are feeling. No one else can do a better job. If people with pain feel that others do not believe them, they become upset and possibly stop reporting their pain accurately. This only makes controlling the pain more difficult.

It usually takes time to get pain under control since pain medicines take time to build up in the bloodstream. The doctor may have to try different medicines or amounts to see what works best. Things you can do on your own for pain also take time to learn. Do not give up just because complete pain control does not happen immediately. Remember, most cancer pain can eventually be controlled.

Pain

93

It is also important to know that pain is not always caused by a tumor. When the person with pain feels something new, many think, "It is the cancer growing. This is a bad sign." However, the pain might not be from the cancer at all. For example, treatments change tissues. Tissues shrink and swell, and this can cause pain. Weight loss or gain also changes tissues and muscles, which can cause pain. Many things can cause new aches and pains in addition to the growth of cancer itself.

How doctors control cancer pain

Physicians who treat cancer pain use the 3-Step Analgesic Ladder for Cancer Pain Management that was developed by the World Health Organization.

These steps are listed in the picture on this page. Doctors usually start pain treatment as low as possible on the ladder and gradually work up until pain control is achieved.

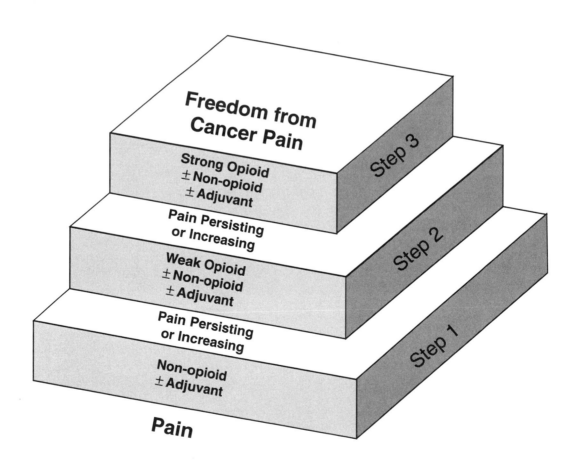

How the pain ladder works

Step 1 for Mild Pain—Nonopioid

The World Health Organization developed a short guide for physicians on managing cancer pain. They outlined an analgesic ladder to show what medicines should be used for mild pain. Nonopioids are mild pain relievers. They are also called:

1. Analgesics: Examples are acetaminophen or Tylenol™.

2. Nonsteroidal anti-inflammatory medicines: Examples are aspirin and ibuprofen (Motrin™ or Advil™).

3. Adjuvants: These medicines treat specific pain and ease other types of symptoms. Examples are antidepressants such as Elavil™, anticonvulsants such as Tegretol™ or Dilantin™, antinausea medicines, and antianxiety medicines such as Xanax™, Valium™, Ativan™, and Atarax™ or Vistaril™.

Step 2 for Moderate Pain—Weak Opioid

If Step 1 drugs do not work, or if the pain is rated as moderate pain, the next step on the ladder shows what medicines should be used. Weak opioids are stronger pain relievers. They are often prescribed to be taken with a nonopioid medicine such as those listed above. Examples of weak opioids are Codeine™, Darvon™ or Darvocet™, and Wygesic™. Stronger medicines in this category include Tylox™, Percocet™, and Percodan™.

Step 3 for Severe Pain—Strong Opioid

The last step on the ladder describes what category of medicines should be used to control severe pain. A strong opioid can be short acting or long acting. Morphine and Numorphan™ are two examples of strong opioids that last 3 to 4 hours. Methadone™ is also a strong opioid giving 4 to 6 hours of pain relief. These medicines are also available in 12-hour release pills.

Your goals are to:

call for help during two different types of emergencies: the experience of severe pain and reactions to pain medicines,

call for help during regular office hours,

make the best use of pain medicines,

understand the medication plan,

ask about changing pain prescriptions when needed,

manage side effects of pain medicines, and

do things on your own to prevent and control pain.

When To Get Professional Help

The first question you should ask is whether professional help is needed because of severe pain. Signs and symptoms listed below indicate that pain is out of control.

In case of an emergency

Call the doctor or nurse if any of the following conditions exist:

➤ **Unable to get up or walk because of pain.** A tumor can press on a nerve and cause severe pain, especially when the person moves. Swelling or inflammation around a tumor can push on tender tissues or nerves. In these examples, persons with cancer feel severe pain, usually complain, and are not able to get up from lying down or to walk without help.

➤ **Unable to sleep because of pain.** Not sleeping well because of discomfort, aches, and pains is a sure sign that something needs to be done to increase comfort.

➤ **Crying and upset about feeling pain.** Look for physical responses to pain: tears, closed eyes, knitted eyebrows, wrinkled forehead, grimaced face, clenched fists, or a stiffened trunk (chest and back), which is held rigidly and moved slowly. When this happens, or when the person complains about severe pain, call the doctor or nurse for help immediately.

➤ **Unwilling to move or muscles are very tense when moving.** Even if he or she does not complain and tries to act as if nothing is wrong, watch how easily he or she moves. People in pain move with great difficulty, do not try to move, and do not do normal everyday things like get dressed or get out of bed.

➤ **A bone sticks out in an unusual way.** Bones can break or fracture more easily as a person gets older. Bone cancer also increases the risk of a fracture. If a bone sticks out in a new way, report this, even if pain does not immediately follow this event.

➤ **Decreased appetite because of pain.** Watch for a sudden decrease in appetite. Although appetite is changed by many other factors, do not rule out aches and pains as the cause of less appetite.

➤ **Less desire to visit with family and friends because of pain.** Pain or discomfort can reduce the desire to visit with family and friends. Withdrawing from normal activities may also be a sign of depression or sadness.

➤ **Actions to take care of "breakthrough pain" are not working and pain continues to be a problem in between doses of long-acting medicines (6 to 12 hours relief expected).** "Breakthrough pain" is pain that breaks through the relief achieved by the regularly scheduled, around-the-clock medicines. The pain occurs in between the scheduled times for giving the pain medicine.

Know the following facts before you call
about an emergency because of severe pain

1. How long has the pain been a problem?

2. Where is it located? Is it in more than one area?

3. How severe is the pain? Ask the person to use any number from 0 to 10 to describe or rate the pain, where 0 = none, 5 = moderate, and 10 = worst ever.

4. Is the pain sharp and stabbing or dull and aching?

5. Does the pain burn or feel like an electric shock?

6. Is there any numbness or tingling?

7. How much has this pain interfered with doing normal activities?

8. Describe any prescriptions for pain:

> Name of medicine(s)
> How much time should go by between doses?
> How many pills can be taken at one time?
> How many doses were taken in the last 2 days?
> How long do they take to work?
> How much relief do they give?
> How long does this relief last?

9. What other medicines have been taken or what else has been done to relieve the pain? What were the results?

Here's an example of what you might say when calling

"I am Mary Smith, wife of John Smith. My husband sees Dr. Harvey. The home care plan for pain said I should call if he complains that his pain is getting worse. This morning he refused to get out of bed because his leg hurt so badly up at the hip, and it hurts even if he tries to move just a little in bed. He said his pain is an "8" and is sharp. At 6 a.m. he took two Percocets™ but didn't feel any better. The next time for his medicine isn't until noon. We tried a heating pad, but it didn't help."

When to get immediate help for effects of pain medicines

A drug reaction or narcotic overdose is a different type of emergency related to pain control. If the person with cancer is allergic to pain medicines, or the pain medicines are too strong, professional help is needed. Call the doctor or nurse immediately if any of the following symptoms occur when taking pain medicines:

➤ **Hallucinations (hearing or seeing things that are not there)**

➤ **Ringing or buzzing in the ears**

➤ **Confusion or being "out of it"**

➤ **Great trouble waking up even when others try to wake the person**

➤ **Severe trembling, uncontrolled muscle movements, or convulsions (seizures)**

➤ **Unable to hold in urine or stool when this was not a problem in the past**

➤ **Unable to urinate despite feeling the need to urinate**

➤ **Nausea or vomiting with no relief**

➤ **Hives, itching, skin rash, or swelling of the face**

Know the following facts before you call about an emergency caused by pain medicines

1. What pain medicine was taken over the last few days?

2. How much medicine was taken?

3. How often was it taken?

Most of the symptoms on this "call now" list indicate that a drug reaction is causing a problem with the central nervous system, the gastrointestinal tract, the urinary tract, or the skin and that the body's normal functioning is severely impaired. Either the medicine is too strong or there is an uncommon allergic reaction.

Side effects like those on this list demand immediate action. When you call and report these symptoms, the doctor or nurse will most likely want to see the person with cancer right away, or they will send emergency help to you. After evaluating what is happening, they can give medicines to clear any drugs out of the body. They can also prescribe other ways to calm the central nervous system and reverse an allergic reaction.

Problems with drug reactions are not that common. When they do happen, it is important to get help right away.

When symptoms are not an emergency, but should be reported

Some symptoms are not considered to be an emergency but should still be reported during regular office hours. Call the doctor or nurse if any of the following conditions exist:

➤ **No relief after taking pain medicine three times, as prescribed.** Call and discuss the pain problem with the doctor or nurse.

➤ **Some pain relief, but there is still significant pain after 1 or 2 days since starting the medicine, changing the way it is taken, or changing the amount taken.** The physician or nurse needs to re-evaluate the amount or type of pain medicine prescribed.

➤ **A new type of pain, pain in new locations, or new pain when moving or sitting.** Report pain in new locations. New pains may need to be evaluated before the next regularly scheduled clinic visit.

➤ **Numbness, tingling, or burning sensations that are new.** They can signal an early problem with the nervous system or with the amount of medicine being taken. Report these immediately so that the doctor or nurse can locate what is causing it and make the necessary changes in the treatment plan. These types of pain may need to be treated with medicines other than commonly prescribed drugs and analgesics. Reporting these sensations can help the doctor or nurse understand that these pains are different from other pains reported in the past. When a tumor invades nerves, there might be a feeling of numbness, tingling, burning, or a short electrical shock. Low doses of antidepressants can help relieve these problems, help sleep, and even readjust chemicals in the spinal cord, which add up to better control of pain.

➤ **Medicines for "breakthrough pain" are used more than three times a day in addition to the regular pain medicines.** Breakthrough pain is when pain happens in between the scheduled times to give the pain medicine. Report whether taking regularly scheduled doses, such as every 4 hours, does not hold back the pain. The doctor may change the medicine schedule or may prescribe extra doses to be given "as needed" or "give prn" (which mean the same thing) when breakthrough pain happens.

➤ **Tremors or involuntary jerking motions while awake or asleep.** These motions can indicate a need for the doctor to adjust the pain medication.

What You Can Do To Help

If you decide that a pain problem is not an emergency and that a drug reaction has not happened, there are five things you can do to solve a problem with cancer pain:

make the best use of medicines,

understand the medication plan,

ask about changing pain prescriptions,

manage common side effects of pain medicine, and

prevent and control pain on your own.

Make the best use of medicines

If the pain is not an emergency, but the person needs medicine on a regular basis, <u>be sure you are using the pain medicine correctly and preventing pain before it becomes severe.</u>

➤ **Give the pain medicine at regular times, as prescribed by the doctor.** When pain occurs regularly and not just once or twice a day, <u>give the pain medicine on a consistent schedule to keep enough medicine in the bloodstream to keep the pain away.</u> Encourage the patient not to wait too long to take it.

For example, suppose the pain medicine is prescribed "every 4 to 6 hours as needed." You can give pain medicine anytime after 4 hours. But do not wait longer than 6 hours because the pain may become so bad that the prescribed amount will not give full relief.

➤ **Give the pain medicine before the pain builds up.** When pain occurs regularly and not just once or twice a day, pain control is more difficult. It also takes longer to achieve control if pain is allowed to build to a severe level. If you do nothing else, <u>give the pain medicine on a regular basis</u>. People need to take pain medicine to avoid a pain crisis just like diabetics need to take insulin to avoid a "sugar" crisis.

<u>Taking the medicine with the same amount of hours between doses prevents peaks and valleys and keeps a steady supply of the medicine in the body</u>. You may even find that you can decrease the amount of medicine given, because the person with pain is more confident that pain can be controlled.

➤ **Continue to give the pain medicine during the night.** Try not to go longer than 8 to 10 hours without giving medicine during the night, unless the person is taking a medicine like MS Contin™ (a time-released capsule), prescribed to be given every 12 hours. <u>Too much time between doses means that the amount of medicine in the body keeps dropping and the level of pain increases</u>. The person with cancer will then need more of the medicine to return to the right level because he or she started below the "normal" medicine level where good pain control was achieved. Giving a dose of pain medicine in the middle of the night helps you to prevent what is called "breakthrough pain."

➤ **Do not stop the pain medicine suddenly if it has been taken for a number of weeks.** If pain medicine is stopped suddenly, the body almost gets a shock. It expects a steadier flow of these medicines into the bloodstream. Withdrawal symptoms can occur in the same way that withdrawal occurs if one suddenly stops smoking cigarettes or drinking coffee. Increasing the length of time between doses and taking lower doses of the pain medicine lets the body be weaned away from the medicines in a gentle manner. The discomfort of withdrawal, such as shakiness or headache, is less likely if the pain medicine is stopped slowly over a few days and under the direction of a physician.

Doing these things also helps to relieve other problems that can increase pain, such as muscle tension, lack of sleep, and emotional distress.

In addition, if you cannot answer the following five questions, then ask your doctor or nurse and learn the answers.

1. What if the medicine wears off and pain returns, but it is too early for the next pain medicine?

2. If the pain is not gone and the pain medicine is taken as prescribed or taken as early as allowed, can more medicine be taken or must we call the doctor?

3. What should I do if pain wakes him or her up at night?

4. What if a dose is accidentally skipped?

5. Is this a medicine that we can crush or have the pharmacist mix in a liquid so it's easier to swallow?

   Some medicine, such as MS Contin™, should not be crushed because all the medicine will be absorbed at one time. This could be dangerous when the purpose of the medicine is to be delivered in a time-released fashion.

Understand the medication plan

Understanding how and when the doctor and nurse want you to give pain medicines is the key to successful pain control and prevention. There are three different plans to follow, and you can ask which one you are on.

Plan 1: Take medicine as needed

➤ **Know when to give a medicine that is prescribed as "give as needed" or "give prn."** Pain medicines can be ordered "as needed." For example, the bottle may be labeled "take every 3 to 4 hours as needed" or "take every 6 hours as needed." This means that people with cancer can decide when to take the medicine but should not take it more frequently than the lowest number of hours listed on the instruction label. If they need the medicine before this lowest number, they should discuss the problem with a doctor or nurse. Maybe the dose is not high enough. Maybe the medicine needs to be combined with another one, such as with Tylenol™ or aspirin, to prevent the pain.

For example, if the prescription is to "take every 3 to 4 hours as needed," people with pain can take the medicine every 3 hours and do so consistently, especially if the pain starts to come back 3 hours after the last dose. Writing down the times that the person with cancer takes pain medicine helps the doctor or nurse to understand what is happening. They can then see that the medicine is being taken every 3 hours—morning, afternoon, evening, and night—and that the person with cancer is not waiting for 4 hours to pass before the next dose. This information is important to tell the doctors and nurses.

Taking medicine "as needed" also means that the person can take a dose and then wait to take another one until they feel the first inkling of pain or before they begin an activity that stimulates the pain problem. For example, some people learn exactly what brings on their pain, such as bending over the stove while cooking or bending over the dryer while laundering. Taking pain medicine before these activities and 3 hours afterwards prevents the pain that could follow bending and exercising.

Plan 2: Take medicine with equal number of hours between doses

➤ **Know when to give a medicine ordered for a certain number of times per day, such as 2, 4, or 6 times a day.** If the medicine is ordered for a certain number of times per day (not for a certain number of hours), then start with the time that he or she wakes up and divide the 24-hour day into equal spaces. For example, if a medicine is ordered as "take twice a day" and the person is usually awake at 9:00 am, then give a dose at 9:00 am and again at 9:00 pm. The times do not have to be exactly right, but you should try to divide the day into even sections. Some examples of dividing the 24-hour day are:

If the dose is ordered as "take 4 times a day," and the person awakens at 9:00 am, then make sure that a dose is taken at 9:00 am, 3:00 pm, 9:00 pm, and 3:00 am, or sometime in the middle of the night.

OR

If the dose is ordered as "take 6 times a day," and the person awakens at 9:00 am, then give the pain medicine at 9:00 am, 1:00 pm, 5:00 pm, 9:00 pm, and during the night at about 1:00 am and 5:00 am.

Plan 3: Take extra medicine when pain breaks through before the next medicine is due

➤ **Treat "breakthrough pain" to prevent its return.** Breakthrough pain is pain or discomfort that happens before it is time for the next dose. Usually, there is a prescription just for when this happens, or the doctor may advise the person with cancer to take an analgesic medicine if pain comes back too soon but it is not time to take the strongest pain medicine itself.

If "breakthrough pain" happens for the first time, make sure that the person is taking pain medicines as frequently as ordered. Sometimes taking the pain medicine more consistently (the same number of hours between doses) and more frequently (for example, if ordered every 4 to 6 hours, then take every 4 hours) around the clock prevents breakthrough pain.

Ask the doctor about changing pain prescriptions, times, and doses

If the person with cancer is taking the medicine as prescribed and the person is still feeling significant pain or is really bothered by the side effects from the current medicine, ask the doctor if there are other medicines or ways to take them that might help more.

➤ **Ask about increasing the amount of medicine.** Sometimes, there is just too little medicine in the body to prevent pain. If so, the doctor may increase the pain medicine by small amounts until the right amount is discovered.

➤ **Ask about shortening the time between doses of pain medicine.** Perhaps the right amount of pain medicine is not kept in the bloodstream because the pain medicine isn't taken often enough. If so, then the doctor may shorten the time between doses to increase the level of the medicine in the body. Talk to the doctor before shortening time between doses. Be sure to say what time the pain medicine was taken and what time (how many hours) the pain returned.

Pain

➤ **Ask about taking short-acting or immediate-release narcotics in between long-acting (time-release) narcotic orders (such as taking immediate-release morphine for "breakthrough pain").** Breakthrough pain means that pain occurs before the next pain pill or shot is due. This can happen even when someone is taking a narcotic that is in a time-released capsule and is good for many hours, such as up to 12 hours. Doctors and nurses who know the latest information on pain control also know that faster-acting narcotics can be ordered to stop breakthrough pain. However, the long-acting dose of narcotic has to be increased if the breakthrough pain occurs more than twice. Some people need to have their narcotic dose (the long-acting pill) almost doubled to prevent breakthrough pain from happening again.

Ask about giving the same medicine in a new form or about using a new technique to give the medicine

An example of a new technique is giving medicine through an intravenous (IV) line that you can take care of at home. There are many new ways to take narcotics and other medicines that relieve pain. Here are some of the different ways that pain medicine can be given:

➤ **Liquid pain medicine.** If people with cancer cannot eat solid foods, they may have trouble swallowing pills. Some pain medicines are available in liquid form. A pharmacist can also mix a liquid syrup with one or more pain medicines in it, which can be given with a measuring spoon.

➤ **Skin patches.** A recent invention is the "transdermal" skin patch, which is placed on the body (chest or back) and delivers a medicine through the skin for up to 72 hours. There are also pills that give pain relief for a long time, such as 12-hour, time-released capsules of morphine.

➤ **Rectal suppositories.** Pain medicine also comes in rectal suppositories. Once placed in the body, they melt and are absorbed into the body.

➤ **Single injections into muscles.** Pain medicine can be received by injection into the muscle or just under the skin. If the idea of a needle scares the person with cancer, very short needles can be used. Many people learn to give shots to family members or friends.

➤ **Subcutaneous (SubQ) needles attached under the skin for 3 days.** A small needle can be placed just under the skin (called subcutaneous or SubQ) by health care workers. Medicine is injected through this line every few hours by a family member.

These lines can be hooked to pumps, which deliver the medicine at regular times. The needle has to be changed and reinserted at a new site every few days by a nurse.

➤ **IV lines into large arm veins.** You may have heard of Hickmans™, Broviacs™, or catheters (sometimes called PICC lines—peripheral inserted central catheters). These are all placed into large arm veins. The tubing comes outside of the skin a few inches, and medicine is given much like with an IV line. The dressings are changed by nurses at the clinic or at home. Lines can even be placed around the spinal column to deliver pain medicine directly to the spinal fluid, if necessary.

➤ **Epidural catheters near the spine.** Anesthesiologists can put epidural catheters near the spine to deliver medicines, and family members can give medicines through these.

➤ **Implanted ports under the skin.** Implanted ports are another new way to get medicine into a large vein in the chest. These ports are about 1 inch wide and 1 inch deep, circular, and metal. They are usually surgically placed under the skin of the upper chest, and a nurse can find its exact placement by gently pushing on the skin and feeling the small round disc. Then the nurse cleans the skin there with Betadine™ (a brown cleaning solution) and can draw blood from the site and can give medicine into the port which flows into the vein.

➤ **IV infusing pumps attached to implanted ports.** There are also small, portable pumps with IV lines that can be carried on a belt. They are battery run and can deliver the medicine evenly day and night. Home health nurses or home IV nurses give medicines through this and teach how to care for the pump and the line. Some patients give themselves medicine through these lines as well. When the person with cancer gives the medicine, we refer to this as patient-controlled analgesia (PCA).

Ask about adding other medicines

The doctor may combine several types of pain medicine that work in different ways to give relief. For example, an antianxiety or antidepressant medicine can be added to decrease emotional tension, which, in turn, improves pain control.

➤ **Ask about changing pain medicines.** If many of these suggestions were tried, and pain persists, it is time for the patient, caregiver, and health care staff to discuss another pain medication plan.

➤ **Ask about the use of radiation therapy for pain.** Sometimes radiation is prescribed to shrink a tumor that is causing pain. Treatments usually are given daily, lasting from a few days up to 4 or 5 weeks to help control pain caused by a tumor.

Pain

➤ **Ask about being referred to a pain clinic to be seen by specialists in pain management.** University and large hospitals have special clinics to evaluate and treat chronic pain. Most pain clinics require that a doctor refer you to them and send the medical chart to their clinic staff.

Doctors, nurses, counselors, and pharmacists at a pain clinic know a lot about special problems with pain. They are interested in helping you solve your pain problem. For example, an anesthesiologist can give a nerve block that stops a feeling of pain for a short time until other methods are prescribed, or the nerve block can be given to last a long time.

Another advantage of a pain clinic is that the staff there might prescribe a combination of two or three medicines that relieve different types of pain.

If there is no pain clinic at your local hospital, you can ask the doctors there to refer the person with cancer to a pain clinic at another hospital. You can also call the pain clinic and ask how referrals are handled.

Manage the more common side effects of pain medicine

Not all people react the same way to pain medicines. However, certain side effects are very common. Watch for these and deal with them early.

➤ **Prevent constipation with diet, liquids, stool softeners, and laxatives.** Narcotics are dehydrating. They take water out of the stools, which results in constipation. Stool softeners are pills that put the water back into the stool, making it less hard and easier to pass. Some people take one or two stool softeners in the morning and one or two at bedtime to prevent this problem.

If stool softeners and laxatives do not work and the person with cancer has not had a bowel movement in 2 to 3 days, give a product that is purely a laxative, such as Milk of Magnesia™. You may have to increase the number of stool softeners and stimulants taken every day. Some people add a mild laxative to the medicine schedule and give one every other day. Others give a mild enema. See the home care plan for Constipation, which describes different types of enemas and how to give them.

Another way to prevent constipation is to serve food with high fiber content, such as prunes, fresh fruit and vegetables, or bran. These add bulk to what is inside the intestines and attract water back into the intestines, which softens the stool. Also, offer fluids—as much as 8 to 10 glasses a day.

➤ **Avoid constipating foods such as cheese or chocolate.**

➤ Relieve a dry mouth with crushed ice, hard candy, and frequent rinses with water or products that do not contain alcohol.

➤ Relieve painful dry nasal passages by humidifying the air or breathing in warm moisture from a sink full of warm water.

➤ Avoid an upset stomach by taking medicine with food, unless instructed otherwise by the pharmacist.

➤ Expect drowsiness for a few days when pain medicine is started or increased. If sleepiness increases just after starting or increasing pain medicine, wait about 3 days. Sometimes sleepiness happens because a person is finally getting pain relief and needs to catch up on missed rest, or the body needs time to adjust to new medicines or doses. If sleepiness is a concern, offer beverages with caffeine in them, if allowed, but discourage driving a car or operating power tools. Narcotics slow the responses in somewhat the way alcohol does. Therefore, postpone activities requiring fast reactions for safety's sake. If the drowsiness lasts longer than a week, contact the doctor so it can be evaluated and corrected. Finally, if drowsiness is extreme and you cannot awaken the person, call the doctor or nurse immediately.

Prevent and control pain on your own

There are many things you can do on your own to help prevent and control pain:

Managing pain medicine

➤ Set an alarm as a reminder to take pain medicine. This reminds you to give the pain medicine or reminds the person with cancer to take the medicine.

➤ Use a medicine tray with slots for time of day to hold the medicines. These are plastic boxes with squares for each day of the week and slots for dose times. Many people fill the box for the whole week. If you are having trouble reading labels, remembering to give pain medicine, or following the dose schedule, get someone else to fill up the medicine tray. You can also use an egg carton and mark each slot with the name of the day of the week and the time that the pain medicine is to be given that day.

➤ Telephone the pharmacy before going to fill the pain prescription. Some pharmacies do not carry all pain medicines. They may have to special order it or send you to another store.

➤ Use the same pharmacy, if possible. If you use the same pharmacists, they will understand what the medication plan is, how it is working, and have suggestions on how to handle side

Pain

effects. They will also know what pain medicines to keep on hand and can answer many of your questions about the medicines.

➤ **Keep at least a 3-day supply of pain medicine.** Call the doctor for a new prescription before the last pain medicine is given. If it is the end of the week, you should have at least a 5-day supply. If you are planning to be out of town, be certain to have a sufficient supply until your planned return.

Helping to control pain

➤ **Use warm showers, baths, hot water bottles, or warm wash-cloths.** Heat relaxes the muscles and gives a sense of comfort. Do not set heating pads on high because they can burn the skin. Do not place them over or near areas where radiation marks are on the skin, even when radiation treatments are finished.

➤ **Use cool cloths or ice.** Cooling the skin and muscles can soothe pain, especially pain that comes from inflammation or swelling. For example, many people like using a cool washcloth on their forehead when they have a headache.

➤ **Position the person carefully with pillows and soft seat cushions.**

➤ **Massage sore spots, such as neck and shoulders.**

➤ **Avoid lifting or straining.**

➤ **Encourage him or her to use deep breathing exercises.** Deep breathing slowly and quietly helps the mind and body to relax and helps decrease pain. Use tape recordings or learn simple methods from books on relaxation. Ask the health care team about these techniques, or read the home care plan for Coping with Anxiety to learn more about relaxation.

➤ **Distract the person with pleasant, involving activities.** Doing such activities takes the mind off of pain. Different people are distracted by different activities. One person may be distracted by watching television or going through a catalog. Another may be distracted by listening to music or visiting with friends. See the home care plan for Maintaining Positive Experiences for additional ideas.

➤ **Ask for help with tasks.** Now is the time for both you and the patient not to overdo it. So get others to lend a hand. Do not be shy about asking for help! It is part of your job as a caregiver to get help when you need it.

➤ **Do activities when feeling most comfortable.** Plan activities when the person with pain is feeling best and is most awake. This might be a few days after a new pain medicine is started or after the dose was increased.

➤ **Keep a diary, rate the pain, and note what makes it worse or better.** A diary can help you tell the doctors and nurses how well the pain treatments are working and can help you judge what progress is being made at home. Writing down what makes the pain worse or better helps you and the person with cancer think clearly about your plan to solve and prevent this problem. Also, keep track of the times, amounts, and names of pain medicines given. If you bring this diary with you to doctor appointments, it helps the staff understand what you are doing, and this helps them make recommendations about treatments.

➤ **Avoid stressful events when possible.** Emotional stress and anxiety increase pain. If you can cancel certain events that are stressful, do so. A "bad atmosphere" is not something your family member or friend needs to struggle with now. See the home care plans on Coping with Anxiety and Coping with Depression for ways to control emotional stress.

➤ **Consider going to a cancer patient support group meeting or educational session in your area.** Many persons with cancer enjoy these, and family and friends are welcome. To find out where and when local support groups meet, look in the telephone book. Usually the phone book has a large section called Guide to Human Services. Cancer support groups are listed under Cancer. Groups for family and friends who help anyone with a chronic illness are listed under Caregivers.

You can also ask nurses, doctors, or social workers about local support groups. The local office of the American Cancer Society often has lists of support groups. Their number is in the white pages of the phone book. You can also call the hospice program in your area. This number is in the yellow pages under Hospice or Home Health Care. If you are not successful, call the Cancer Information Hot Line at the National Cancer Institute: 1-800-4-CANCER.

Possible Obstacles

Think about ideas or attitudes that could prevent you from carrying out any of these strategies.

Here are some common obstacles that have stopped others from giving (or taking) pain medicines

1. Either you or the person with cancer says, "I'm afraid of addiction."

   Response: <u>People who take narcotics for pain rarely become addicted</u>. In fact, if their pain is treated effectively, it decreases the risk of addiction.

Pain

People who are "addicts" take drugs for a "high" or an altered state of mind. People who take narcotics for cancer pain take them to get relief from physical pain. People who are *not* addicts before they take narcotics for cancer pain do *not* become addicts later. Remember that the medicine is being used for pain control and not for a psychological "high." Pain medicines can be stopped in such a way that the person does not have the side effects of withdrawal.

Even if you understand that your friend or family member is not addicted, others may not. Do not spend a lot of your energy changing their minds. Tell them that this medicine is part of the medical treatment and absolutely crucial to the person's quality of life and ability to do what is most important to them.

2. "I want to 'save' the pain medicine and give it when the pain is severe."

Response: Taking pain medicine for mild discomfort now does not affect how well it will work in the future or when the pain gets worse. Don't hold back the pain medicines you take today in order to save up if more pain medicine is needed later. In fact, it takes more medicine to treat the pain that is uncontrolled than it does to prevent pain from building up.

People do sometimes need to increase their doses of pain medicine. Their need for more medicine does not mean that they are becoming "immune" to pain medicines or that they need more and more medicine to control the same level of pain. These people need more medication because the pain has changed. Actually, there is no real limit for most of the drugs to the dose a person can take. A few do have upper limits. If the person with pain reaches that limit, the doctor can change to a different pain medicine. The doctor knows when it is right to change a medicine.

If pain is controlled now, you and the person with pain should be less worried about controlling it later because you know that the medicines do work. Also, taking enough medicine now helps the person with pain to relax and to preserve his or her strength.

3. The person with pain feels that "No one wants to hear about my pain."

   Response: The person with pain should understand that family and friends may seem uninterested because they feel helpless. Doctors and nurses who specialize in pain, such as those in a pain clinic or hospice, do understand pain problems. Talk to them if you are feeling alone with these problems.

4. "He doesn't want to take any morphine because that means he's dying. Only people who are close to death take that drug."

   Response: Morphine is not reserved for the dying. It is an effective medicine for many types of cancer pain. Taking it does not mean a person is near death. It is also used to control chronic pain during earlier phases of the disease. Some people go back to work and do their regular daily activities because the morphine is so effective. It lets them return to pain-free lives.

Think of *other* obstacles that could interfere with carrying out your plan

What additional road blocks could get in the way of doing the things recommended in this home care plan? For example, will the person with cancer cooperate? Will other people help? How will you explain your needs to other people? Do you have the time and energy to carry out the plan?

You need to develop plans for getting around these road blocks. Use the four COPE ideas (creativity, optimism, planning, and expert information) in developing your plans. See the chapter on Solving Home Care Problems at the beginning of the book for a discussion of how to use the four COPE ideas in overcoming your obstacles.

Carrying Out and Adjusting Your Plan

Checking on results

Keep track of the pain level. You can do this by asking the person you are caring for to tell you how severe the pain is. Use the same terms each time you do this so that you can compare one time with another. This helps you to evaluate how effective your pain control program is and to notice changes. For example, you might want to use the words "worst ever," "severe," "bad," "moderate," "mild," and "none at all" each time. The person who is telling you about the pain can choose which word fits best or even say it is between the words (for example, "it is between severe and bad"). Another way to do this is to think of a 10-inch ruler, where 10 is the worst pain ever, 0 is no pain, and 5 is moderate pain. Then the person can give you a number to fit his or her pain.

If these ratings are to be meaningful, it is essential that the person with pain understand that you fully accept his or her ratings. Pain can be judged only by the person who has it. <u>The person with cancer has to feel that you trust and accept what is said about pain—or he or she won't cooperate or will give incorrect information</u>.

If your plan doesn't work

If problems with pain are getting worse, review When To Get Professional Help. If you decide to call the doctor or nurse, tell them what was done to deal with pain and discuss what else could be done.

If you do not think that you need to talk with a doctor or nurse immediately or during regular office hours about pain, then ask yourself if you are doing everything you can to make the best use of medicines and to control pain on your own. Review this home care plan to be sure you are doing everything you can to deal with this problem.

Remember: <u>Cancer pain can be very well controlled. Do not accept anything less than the best pain control</u>.

If you feel that the medical staff is not listening to your concerns or is not able to give adequate pain control, you can ask them to refer you to a cancer pain specialist. These are physicians who specialize in cancer pain and can usually be found at cancer centers, or they may be local physicians who are involved in hospice care. A book for physicians which is highly recommended by cancer pain specialists is described here:

The *Handbook of Cancer Pain Management* is written by cancer pain specialists for physicians.

The handbook explains the steps on the "Analgesic Ladder," lists the drugs that doctors can prescribe at each step, and explains how to manage possible side effects. It was written in 1988 by pain specialists from a number of different organizations and is published by the Wisconsin Cancer Pain Initiative program. It can be ordered by calling 608-262-0978. There is a cost for the handbook. Bulk prices are also available, depending on volume and use.

Only 36 pages long, the *Handbook of Cancer Pain Management* is pocket-sized and includes six appendices: Narcotic Equivalency Index, Opioid Preparations, Continuous Opioid Infusions, the World Health Organization's Analgesic Ladder, Pain Scale for Children, and Licensing and Prescribing Information.

Problems with Veins

Overview of the
Home Care Plan for Problems with Veins

Understanding the Problem

Importance of protecting veins

What happens when veins are injured

After treatment, most people's veins return to normal

There are ways to get blood and to give intravenous medicines without sticking the arm every time

When To Get Professional Help

Symptoms that require professional help

Facts to know when you call

What to say when you call

What You Can Do To Help

How to prepare veins and skin for needle sticks

How to limit discomfort and anxiety during needle sticks

Learn about alternatives to needle sticks into veins and for giving intravenous medicines

Possible Obstacles

"The staff didn't say anything about ports or catheters, so I assumed they shouldn't be used."

"There's always been trouble with needle sticks."

Carrying Out and Adjusting Your Plan

Keep track of vein problems

Report unresolved problems to medical staff

(Topics with an arrow in front of them are actions you can take or symptoms you can look for.)

Problems with Veins

[The information in this home care plan fits most situations, but yours may be different.

If the doctor or nurse tells you to do something else, follow what they say. If you think there may be a medical emergency, see page 116.]

Understanding the Problem

Many chemotherapy treatments are injected into veins, and veins are used to obtain samples for blood and diagnostic tests. It is therefore important to protect the veins of anyone with cancer. Some people have a difficult time having their blood drawn or having needles put into their veins because the veins become sore or are hard to find and use. In some instances, people may also become anxious about these "needle sticks" (venipuncture). This home care plan explains what you can do to minimize these problems as well as some new ways to get blood or give drugs without needle sticks in the arms.

After treatments are over, most people's veins return to normal. In some cases, veins can be damaged for a long time. Chemotherapy can cause sclerosis of the veins, which means they harden and cannot be punctured again.

Needle sticks are, for the most part, unavoidable. You need to help the person with cancer protect their veins and prevent undue anxiety about this procedure, and you should learn about new options to having neeedle sticks in the arm.

Your goals are to:

call for professional help if it is needed,

prepare veins and skin for needle sticks,

limit discomfort or anxiety during needle sticks, and

know about alternatives to needle sticks and the new options for getting drugs that are given into the veins and for getting blood drawn.

Veins

When To Get Professional Help

The first question you should ask is whether you need help from medical professionals.

In case of an emergency

The three problems listed below indicate a serious skin or vein problem. Each needs to be evaluated and handled by a health professional. <u>Call the doctor or nurse if any of the following conditions exist</u>:

➤ **Aching, tenderness, swelling, or redness (particularly a red streak) anywhere on the arm where the needle stick (venipuncture) was done.** Report any of these problems so that the nurse can decide whether the person with cancer needs to come into the clinic to have the arm or vein inspected. These signs might mean that the skin or vein is reacting to the drug. The staff can also tell you over the telephone how to treat the problem, such as by putting ice on the skin or using warm compresses.

➤ **Any drainage, pus, or blisters at the site where a needle stick was done.** Clear or yellow-colored liquid coming from the needle stick site could indicate an infection. Blisters also have fluid in them and should be reported.

➤ **The person is so upset or nervous about "needle sticks" that they consider skipping the treatment or blood draw.** Few people become so anxious about having their blood drawn that it stops them from going to a clinic appointment or visiting the lab. Increasing anxiety about this procedure could lead to someone refusing treatments or blood draws. Professional staff know how to decrease anxiety about venipuncture. <u>Address this problem early to help regain a sense of calmness</u>.

Know the following information before you call

1. When did the skin or vein problem start?

2. Where are the veins that are sore?

3. When was chemotherapy or a blood draw done at the sites that are sore?

4. Is there a dark black or blue bruise?

Here is an example of what you might say when calling

"I am Joan Smith, Harry Smith's wife. My husband is Dr. Harvey's patient. The home care plan on problems with veins says to call if there is swelling anywhere on the arm. The skin is puffy at the injection site. Chemotherapy was given yesterday at 2:00, and he noticed these problems when we got home."

What You Can Do To Help

If the problem is not an emergency, then there are three things you can do to help with sore veins and needle sticks:

prepare veins and skin for needle sticks,

limit discomfort and anxiety during needle sticks, and

learn about alternatives to needle sticks into arm veins.

Prepare skin and veins for needle sticks

There are certain things the person with cancer can do to make the veins dilate so they are easily seen by whomever is going to do the needle stick. Other actions prepare the skin to be stuck by a needle as smoothly as possible.

➤ **Stay warm.** Warmth makes the veins relax and fill up with blood. Sometimes the chemotherapy nurses wrap the arm in a warm, wet cloth a few minutes before an injection. This helps the veins to dilate.

➤ **Eat well the day before the treatment.** Food and fluids help to maintain good blood flow through the veins. On the day of treatment, you should eat and drink normally in the morning unless you are scheduled for tests that require fasting (not eating anything).

➤ **Drink 2 to 3 quarts of liquid every day**, if possible. Fluids dilate or inflate the veins. Blood flows better and the veins are more likely to stick up and be found easily. Drink as much as possible, unless fluids are restricted for other reasons, such as heart disease.

➤ **Take a walk while waiting for chemotherapy or a blood draw.** Walking to the clinic or near the clinic area helps to increase good blood flow and keeps the veins pumped up so they are easier to "stick."

➤ **Exercise the hands and arms at home.** Exercising at home can help make veins bigger. Encourage the person with cancer to squeeze a rubber ball or lift small weights, like cans of soup. He

Veins

or she can do this while talking with family or friends or watching television.

➤ **Use moisturizer lotions.** Apply a favorite lotion, cream, or ointment to the skin from fingertips to elbows. Lotion keeps the skin moisturized, which prevents dryness, cracking, and thickening of the skin. When the skin is dry, it's harder and more painful to puncture with a needle. The best time to apply moisturizers is after your skin has been wet—after bathing, showering, swimming, or doing dishes. Pat your skin almost dry and then apply the lotion. Do this as often as possible, at least four times each day.

Limit discomfort and anxiety during needle sticks

Venipunctures or "needle sticks" make many people anxious, so the person with cancer is not alone. <u>There are several things you can do to help reduce or minimize any anxiety</u>.

➤ **Give antinausea medicines, which also promote relaxation.** Be sure to give antinausea medicines before chemotherapy treatments. Many of these medicines decrease anxiety as a natural side effect.

➤ **Remember and talk about pleasant experiences while waiting.** Have the person with cancer talk and think about pleasant experiences while waiting for treatment or a blood draw. Suggest doing an activity that is involving to take the mind off of the treatments, such as reading an interesting magazine or talking with another patient about something pleasant. Sometimes talking to the nurse about something other than the needle stick can distract him or her.

➤ **Remind the person to look away from the arm.** Many lab workers and nurses distract the person receiving a needle stick by talking with them. Suggest that the person also look somewhere else in the room during the procedure.

➤ **Talk to the doctor and nurse about the anxiety.** The doctor may prescribe a medicine to make the person more relaxed or may recommend a mental health professional to help with these feelings. The home care plan for Coping with Anxiety may also help.

➤ **Practice deep breathing, and use this skill when receiving intravenous treatments or needle sticks.** There are books and tapes that teach deep muscle relaxation. Ask the nurse to recommend a book or tape that has been helpful to other patients. The home care plan on Cancer Pain explains several ways to relax.

➤ **Practice relaxation techniques at home, and then repeat these techniques before and during needle sticks.** Relaxation is a skill and improves with practice. When the person with cancer practices at home, he or she can then use that skill to relax in medical settings. See the home care plan for Coping with Anxiety for ideas about how to become relaxed.

Learn about alternatives to needle sticks into arm veins

If needle sticks are a continuing problem or if the person with cancer is going to be receiving many of them over time, there are other ways to get blood out of the body for routine tests and other ways to get drugs into the body. Three options are available at most large medical centers and have been used by many people with cancer for the last 10 to 20 years.

➤ **Ask about finger sticks for some blood draws.** Sometimes a finger stick—a pin prick on the finger that gives only a drop or two of blood—is all that is needed for certain tests, such as a complete blood count (CBC) or platelet count. Ask your nurse or lab technician if this is an option for the tests that are to be done.

➤ **Ask about intravenous (IV) catheters that connect to large veins.** These catheters are special small, flexible, and sterile tubes that can be put into large blood vessels under the skin. They are the same size as most IV lines. They can be threaded through the skin into a large vein on the chest or threaded up the arm. They can stay in for months and are taped to the chest or arm. These catheters, sometimes called Broviacs™ or Hickmans™, are used to draw blood for lab tests and to inject medicine or drugs used in chemotherapy into a large vein. Some people choose to have these inserted to avoid needle sticks in the arms and hands. The skin around the catheter is easily cleansed, and the site is not noticeable through clothing. If you are interested in finding out more about these options, ask your nurse or doctor about them.

➤ **Ask about permanent ports or blood access devices that can be placed under the skin.** Another way to get drugs into the body without sticking a vein every time is through a permanent port site. These are small (about 1 inch), round metal discs that are placed under the skin, usually on the chest. A small IV line extends from them into a large vein. If you press lightly on the skin, you can feel them, but they are barely visible from the outside. Needles are pushed into the port site and the drug is injected directly into the port that is connected to the large vein. Ask about this option also.

Ask about differences between IV catheters and permanent ports under the skin.

a. How often does the catheter or port need to be flushed to stay open, and who will do this?

Ports need to be flushed only once every 4 weeks if no drugs are given and no blood is taken. The person with cancer can visit a doctor's office or clinic and have this done. It takes 5 minutes. Visiting nurses can also do this at home if it is too hard for the person with cancer to travel. A few persons with cancer learn to do this themselves, but it takes good control of fingers and good vision to do it alone. A needle is used and pushed through the skin to get to the port underneath, but this does not usually hurt.

Intravenous catheters in the chest must be flushed every day to keep them open and available for future use. The dressing around them needs to be changed only three times per week. Again, caregivers and family members can learn to do this, but they must be good with their hands and be able to see well. It's important to plan, in advance, who can change these dressings, clean the skin around it, and flush the catheter every day.

b. How much can a person move and exercise with catheters and ports?

Ports do not prevent athletic exercise. Because the port is under the skin, the person with cancer can swim, play sports, and do any athletic activity that they want.

Catheters hang outside of the body, so swimming and some athletic sports are not advised because the catheter might be pulled out.

c. Will the treatments he or she is receiving be better with catheters or with ports?

Some medical centers require that a catheter be used with certain drugs. People with leukemia, for example, need to have a catheter inserted to receive large amounts of IV fluids and drugs. If you know that the person with cancer might be sent to a different medical center for cancer treatment, ask which option that center prefers to use, and use the one they recommend.

d. Will the catheter or port need more than one opening?

A "double" opening port or catheter lets two different drugs run into a large vein at the same time. A "triple" opening lets three drugs be given at the same time, and so on. They give the person with cancer more treatment options, especially when hospitalized.

Possible Obstacles

Think about what could prevent you from carrying out your plan.

Here are some obstacles that sometimes stop people from carrying out their plan to deal with needle sticks and sore veins

1. "The staff didn't say anything about ports or catheters, so I assumed that they shouldn't be used."

   Response: The staff may not know how upsetting needle sticks are to the person with cancer, so they don't think it is a problem. If it takes three or more attempts to do needle sticks in the arms, you should ask about the availability and advisability of using ports or catheters.

2. "I've had trouble with needle sticks all my life, so nothing can be done."

   Response: Health care staff who give cancer treatments are usually very experienced In doing "needle sticks." They have had special training in how to do this procedure, and they understand how difficult this can be for some people. Therefore, you may find that "needle sticks" in a cancer clinic are much less of a problem than you thought they might be. Health care staff are sensitive to this concern and will suggest ways to make the procedure as easy as possible.

Think of *other* obstacles that could interfere with carrying out your plan

What additional road blocks could get in the way of doing the things recommended in this home care plan? For example, will the person with cancer cooperate? Will other people help? How will you explain your needs to medical staff? Do you have the time and energy to carry out the plan?

You need to develop plans for getting around these road blocks. Use the four COPE ideas (creativity, optimism, planning, and expert information) in developing your plans. See the chapter on Solving Home Care Problems at the beginning of the book for a discussion of how to use the four COPE ideas in overcoming your obstacles.

Veins

Checking on results

Are nurses and laboratory technicians able to find veins for needle sticks? Is the skin near the veins moist and unbruised? Is the person with cancer worried or upset about needle sticks? If there are problems with needle sticks, have alternative ways of drawing blood or giving medicines been considered? If you answer "yes" to these questions, you are meeting your goals and preventing or solving problems with sore veins or needle stick procedures. Keep a close eye on this situation in case it changes. If you answered "no" to any of these questions, then you need to review this home care plan.

If your plan doesn't work

If problems with veins are getting worse, or if the person with cancer is becoming more and more anxious, review What You Can Do To Help in this home care plan. <u>If you have done all that you can, then ask the nurse or doctor about the different options for IV lines or ports on a short- or long-term basis.</u>

Problems with Bleeding

Overview of the
Home Care Plan for Problems with Bleeding

Understanding the Problem

Why chemotherapy increases the risk for bleeding

When To Get Professional Help

Symptoms that require professional help

Facts to know when you call for help

What to say when you call

What You Can Do To Help

How to control bleeding

How to prevent future bleeding

Possible Obstacles

"I need to take aspirin for my arthritis."

Carrying Out and Adjusting Your Plan

Keep track of blood counts and chemotherapy dates to understand
when risk of bleeding is higher

If problems continue, contact medical staff

(Topics with an arrow in front of them are actions you can take or symptoms you can look for.)

Problems with Bleeding

[The information in this home care plan fits most situations, but yours may be different.

If the doctor or nurse tells you to do something else, follow what they say. If you think there may be a medical emergency, see pages 125–126.]

Understanding the Problem

Platelets are made inside the bone marrow and help the blood to clot, or stop flowing. Chemotherapy affects the bone marrow's ability to make platelets, and the number of platelets drops after certain kinds of chemotherapy. As a result, people receiving certain kinds of chemotherapy are at higher risk for unusual bleeding, such as after shaving or brushing their teeth.

When a person is receiving chemotherapy, you should know whether it affects bleeding. If it does, you should know when to get professional help if bleeding occurs, how to spot bleeding in its early stages, how to control bleeding, and how to help prevent it.

Your goals are to:

call when professional help is needed,

control bleeding if it starts, and

prevent future bleeding.

When To Get Professional Help

In case of an emergency

You should urge the person to call the doctor or nurse or make the call yourself if any of the following conditions exist:

➤ **Any unusual or sudden bleeding lasting more than 10 minutes, such as nose bleeds or bleeding gums.** Tiny capillaries are at the end of the blood flow system that branches out through the whole body. Most bleeding that we can see comes from these small blood vessels. The nose and mouth have many of these capillaries near the surface of the skin. These are the easiest places to break open and bleed.

➤ **Vomiting of blood or coffee ground material.** In rare cases, bright red blood can be vomited. Blood in vomit, however, is more likely to be very dark in color and look like coffee grounds. This is blood that has been collecting in the stomach or abdomen because of a bleeding ulcer or sore.

➤ **Blood in the urine. Look for red, pink, or dark urine.** Urine is usually light yellow. It is a brighter yellow when it is more concentrated, for example, when a person is not drinking much fluid. Pink- or red-colored urine indicates a problem with bleeding to the doctor or nurse. A change from yellow to a dark-colored urine should also be reported, although it may not be caused by blood.

➤ **Blood in the stools. Look for red, dark red, or black stools.** Bright red blood around a stool means that blood vessels close to the rectum are open and bleeding. Hemorrhoids can cause this. Dark black or tar-colored stools indicate a bleeding problem higher in the intestinal tract. The blood is older and darker by the time you see a change in the bowel movement.

➤ **Little red or purple spots on the skin or in the mouth, which appear quickly.** Tiny capillaries or blood vessels can open up in areas where they are closest to the skin surface. When they bleed underneath the skin, they leave dots or spots that are red or purple in color. These can be seen in the mouth or on the skin.

➤ **Cough, sputum, or phlegm have blood.** Very small amounts of blood or streaks of blood may appear when the person with cancer coughs up phlegm (a thick, wet discharge produced after coughing). If this happens more than once or if the phlegm is quite bloody, then report it to the doctor.

Know the following facts before you call the doctor or nurse

1. When did this sign of bleeding start?

2. How long did it last?

3. How much was there?

4. Has the person coughed up blood?

5. For women: Is there vaginal bleeding? How heavy is the flow?

6. Is there bleeding anywhere else? Where?

7. What medications were taken recently?

___ Aspirin

___ Ibuprofen™, Motrin™, Advil™

___ Iron

___ Suppositories

___ Chemotherapy (when?)

___ Prednisone™

___ Decadron™

8. Is the person receiving radiation therapy? If yes, where on the body?

9. Did the person with cancer have problems in the past with stomach ulcers or other bleeding problems?

10. When were the last blood counts done, and what were the platelet levels?

Here's an example of what you might say when calling

"I am Jane Smith, Harvey Smith's wife. My husband sees Dr. Jones at the oncology clinic. The home care plan on bleeding says to call if he has a bad nose bleed. He just started chemotherapy this week, and I was worried that the chemotherapy may have caused it."

What You Can Do To Help

If you decide that the bleeding problem is not an emergency, here are two things you can do to solve it:

control the bleeding, and

prevent future bleeding.

Control the bleeding

When bleeding starts, it often flows from tiny capillaries that are near the skin surface, such as from the nose or gums. These capillaries open easily, but they also close easily. Try the following three methods to stop the bleeding:

➤ **Press on the area of bleeding.** Pressing on the skin gives the blood in the capillaries more time to clot. Apply pressure to the skin around the bleeding site for about 4 minutes, using a clean, dry washcloth to maintain the pressure. Do not peek to see if the bleeding has stopped until after 4 minutes. You can also use an elastic bandage or gauze and firmly tape it around the wound, depending on where the bleeding is.

➤ **For nosebleeds, put ice on the nose and press the nose and back of the neck.** Pressing gives more time to stop the bleeding. For a nose bleed, press the nose with a handkerchief or put ice wrapped in a soft cloth over the bridge of the nose for a full 5 minutes and press firmly on the nostrils. Ice makes the capillaries shrink, which helps to control bleeding. Do not check to see if the bleeding has stopped or peek at the nose bleed until after 5 minutes have gone by.

➤ **Tilt head back for nosebleeds, but don't lie down because this causes blood to drip into the throat.** Try not to swallow the blood during a nose bleed.

Prevent bleeding

There are many ways to prevent bleeding and bruising when the platelet count is low.

➤ **Do not use ibuprofen or ibuprofen products** such as Motrin™, Advil™, Naprosyn™, Indocin™, Anaprox™, Clinoril™, Feldene™, or Tolestin™. These drugs prevent the blood from clotting in the normal amount of time. Avoid giving these when platelet counts are low.

➤ **Do not use aspirin or products containing aspirin (ASA, acetylsalicylic acid, or salicylate)** such as Alka Seltzer™, Dristan™, Percodan™, Anacin™, Ecotrin™, Pepto-Bismol™, Ascriptin™, Excedrin™, Sominex™, Bromoseltzer™, Fiorinol™, Vanquish™, Congespirin™, or Midol™. At the drugstore, read the fine print on the label of any analgesic or pain relief pill. It may list aspirin or acetylsalicylic acid as part of the ingredients. This means the pill has aspirin in it. Aspirin makes a person bleed more easily, especially when platelet counts are low. Aspirin is included in many products, such as Alka Seltzer™, so be sure to check the list of ingredients.

➤ **Do give aspirin-free products such as acetaminophen,** Tylenol™, Datril™, or Aspirin-Free Anacin™.

➤ **Do not floss teeth.** This can cut the gums and bleeding may be hard to stop.

➤ **Ask if you can give acetaminophen (Tylenol™) as a substitute for aspirin or ibuprofen.**

➤ **Buy soft toothbrushes or sponge-type toothbrushes.** Gums bleed easily when irritated or scraped. A soft toothbrush treats the gums much more gently so that they are less likely to bleed.

➤ **Encourage rinsing and brushing teeth after eating.** Rinsing helps remove any left-over food, which can build up and start an abscess or sore and make the gums bleed.

➤ **Serve a soft, bland diet, such as soup, pureed meats, mashed potatoes, custards, gelatin, or puddings, if there is mouth soreness.** Soft foods are the least likely to create a cut or scrape in the mouth. Bland, nonspicy foods are also less likely to cause bleeding. Avoid hot temperature foods. Think back to when you burned the top of your mouth on pizza or a grilled cheese sandwich. The skin tore. When the platelets are low, the skin will also bleed if it tears because it was burnt.

➤ **Suggest using petroleum jelly or lip balm but not Vaseline™.**

➤ **Remind the person with cancer to blow the nose gently.** There are many tiny blood vessels in and near the nose that can open up if the nose is blown too forcefully.

➤ **Check that shaving is done only with an electric razor.**

➤ **Limit the use of sharp objects such as knives, scissors, or tools.**

➤ **Avoid situations of potential harm and injury.** When platelet counts are low, it's important to choose options that carry less risk of injury. For example, take a car or bus rather than ride a bicycle or motorcycle. Take an elevator rather than climb stairs. Avoid contact sports. It's easy for small blood vessels to be damaged by bumps or falls.

➤ **Get others to do heavy lifting and strenuous activities.**

➤ **Review ways to avoid constipation.** Straining to move the bowels can cause bleeding, especially around the rectum. See the home care plan for Constipation for more explanation of what to do to avoid constipation.

➤ **Pad the top of the hands with gauze if bumping them is likely to happen.** If bumping the hands happens a lot and bruising occurs, consider taping a small piece of gauze onto the top of the hands as protection. Padding reduces the chance of bruising a vein and opening it up to bleed.

➤ **Do not use rectal thermometers, suppositories, or enemas, or have rectal intercourse.** Anything put into the rectum can tear these delicate tissues, and bleeding can start easily. Rectal intercourse can also cause bleeding.

➤ **Remind women with cancer not to use vaginal douches.**

➤ **Help keep open cuts or scrapes clean to avoid infection.**

➤ **Ask about blood counts.** Ask the staff to explain platelet counts, what makes them go up and down, and what happens to a person with cancer as platelet counts rise and fall. If platelet counts fall very low or if bleeding develops, the doctor may prescribe a platelet transfusion.

Possible Obstacles

Think about what could prevent you from carrying out your plan to control or prevent bleeding.

Here is one obstacle that other people have faced

1. "I need to take aspirin for my arthritis."

    Response: When a person is receiving cancer treatments, especially chemotherapy, it's important *not* to take most arthritic medicines even though they help the arthritis.

They put the person with cancer at risk for bleeding. Discuss this with the doctor and ask about other ways to control arthritis pain.

Think of *other* obstacles that could interfere with carrying out your plan

What additional road blocks could get in the way of doing the things recommended in this home care plan? For example, will the person with cancer cooperate? Will other people help? How will you explain your needs to medical staff? Do you have the time and energy to carry out the plan?

You need to develop plans for getting around these road blocks. Use the four COPE ideas (creativity, optimism, planning, and expert information) in developing your plans. See the chapter on Solving Home Care Problems at the beginning of the book for a discussion of how to use the four COPE ideas in overcoming your obstacles.

Carrying Out and Adjusting Your Plan

Checking on results

Are you getting professional help when it is needed? Are you able to stop the bleeding on your own whenever it starts? Are the skin and mouth as well cared for and protected as they can be? Are other precautions to prevent bleeding being followed?

Keep a close eye on this situation in case it changes. <u>You might want to consider keeping track of blood counts and chemotherapy dates to understand when the risk for bleeding is higher.</u>

If your plan doesn't work

If problems with bleeding are getting worse, then ask yourself if you are doing everything you can to protect the skin against bruises, bumps, or cuts and to encourage good oral hygiene. Also, review When To Get Professional Help in this home care plan. If you call the doctor or nurse, report the facts about the bleeding and what you have done to deal with the problem.

Skin Problems

Overview of the
Home Care Plan for Skin Problems

Understanding the Problem

What causes skin problems

Types of skin problems that happen with chemotherapy and radiation therapy

Almost all skin problems improve after treatments are over

When To Get Professional Help

Symptoms that require professional help

Facts you will need when you call

What to say

What You Can Do To Help

Relieve itching

Prevent dryness and itching

Conceal dark skin, veins, or nails

Treat acne

Limit sweating

Decrease sun sensitivity

Care of skin during and after radiation therapy

Possible Obstacles

"It's only the skin and not the body."

"I'll just have to live with this itching."

"I'm afraid my skin will be fried by radiation therapy."

Carrying Out and Adjusting Your Plan

Keep track of skin problems

If problems persist, get professional help

(Topics with an arrow in front of them are actions you can take or symptoms you can look for.)

Skin Problems

[The information in this home care plan fits most situations, but yours may be different.

If the doctor or nurse tells you to do something else, follow what they say. If you think there may be a medical emergency, see pages 134–135.]

Understanding the Problem

Many people experience changes in their skin during cancer treatments. Sometimes chemotherapy causes skin changes. Some of these are more bothersome than others. The skin can become dry and itchy. Rashes or little sores can appear. Some people sweat more when receiving chemotherapy. Skin, veins, and fingernails may become darker. Chemotherapy may also make the person with cancer more prone to sunburn.

Radiation therapy causes skin problems that can last several weeks after treatments are completed. Typical skin reactions include dryness, itching, and redness. These reactions are confined to the areas where the radiation beam enters or exits the body. Radiation therapy to a warm, moist area, for example, the groin or armpit, is more likely to affect the skin than treatment to a dry area. Most of these reactions go away a few weeks after treatment is finished, but sometimes the treated skin stays dark long after treatment is over.

<u>Some of these skin problems can be eliminated, some can be reduced, and some will not get better until treatments are completed. Almost all skin problems improve after treatments are over.</u>

Your goals are to:

call for help when it is needed,

relieve itching,

prevent dryness,

conceal dark skin, veins, or nails,

treat acne,

limit sweating,

decrease sun sensitivity, and

take care of skin during and after radiation therapy.

When To Get Professional Help

The following signs usually point to a problem with a drug, chemotherapy, an important body organ, an infection, or too much sun.

Call the doctor or nurse if any of the following conditions exist

➤ **Skin gets very rough, red, or painful.** If you see these skin changes, report them. Also report any new drugs or lotions that are being used. Roughness or redness may signal an allergic skin reaction to a new medicine. If chemotherapy was started recently, if the dose was changed, or if new drugs were added to the chemotherapy list, report these medication changes, too. The cause of redness or roughness may also be external, for example, an allergic reaction to a detergent or soap. Therefore, you should also report any new lotions or soaps that the person with cancer is using.

➤ **A cut becomes very red, sore, or swollen.** Report any cuts that are not healing. They may become painful when lightly touched, and the skin around the cut may become shiny, red, and raised. If you act early, you can prevent serious skin infections.

➤ **A rash or hives starts.** These conditions may also suggest a drug reaction or a reaction to food or liquid. If you do not know what caused this skin problem and he or she has no history of rash or hives, then it's best to call.

➤ **Severe itching lasts more than 3 days.** Itching can be a very bothersome side effect of a drug. It can also be caused by the release of chemicals through the skin that the body cannot process—the excess substances get pushed through the pores of the skin.

➤ **Skin is scratched open and looks red.** If itching becomes severe, the person may scratch the skin open and not even realize it. Red and open skin can then become infected.

➤ **Pus comes out of an opening or cut.** Pus usually indicates a skin infection. Pus from any opening should be reported.

➤ **Skin turns yellow.** Color changes on the skin signal that a major organ is not working well. For example, if a person turns yellow, this can mean that the liver is not working correctly.

➤ **Urine becomes the color of tea.** Color changes in the urine are another signal that a major organ is not working well or that some bleeding is occurring higher up in the urinary system.

➤ **Bowel movements are clay-colored.** Clay-colored stool is more white than orange. It is not any shade of brown and signals the release of body chemicals that should not be concentrated in the stool.

➤ **A bruise does not improve in a week.** Bruises that do not heal can mean that the platelet counts are low, and very slow bleeding may still be occurring at the site of the bruise.

Know the answers to the following questions before you call the doctor or nurse

This information will help the doctor or nurse determine the seriousness of the reported skin problems and what to do about them. The underlying cause needs to be understood, if possible, and these questions investigate not only the length and severity of the current problem, but also its origin. Sometimes very subtle information hints at what created the skin problem, for example, whether its cause is external, such as an allergic reaction to a detergent or soap, or internal.

1. When did the problem start?

2. What do you think brought it on?

3. How bad or embarrassing is it?

4. What helps it feel or look better?

5. What is the person's temperature?

6. How long does it take a bruise to go away?

7. If there is a rash, what makes it begin and when does it go away?

8. Are there any cuts that are not healing?

9. If there is itching, where is it and what relieves it?

10. When was the last chemotherapy treatment?

11. What other medicines are being taken?

If a new chemotherapy has been started recently, report this along with the skin problems. Perhaps the problems result from the new drug or other medicine and indicate an allergic reaction. Hives or a red skin rash that is bothersome or itches suggests an allergic reaction. If chemotherapy was started recently, if the dose was changed, or if new drugs were added to the chemotherapy list, report these medication changes. Red, rough, or painful skin usually signals an unusual reaction to a medication.

Here is an example of what you might say when calling

"I am Joan Smith, Harry Smith's wife. My husband is Dr. Harvey's patient. The home care plan for skin problems says that I should call if he scratched his skin open. He's been itching for days, and now the skin on his arm has broken open."

There are seven things you can do to deal with skin problems:

relieve itching,

prevent dryness and itching,

conceal dark skin, veins, or nails,

treat acne,

limit sweating,

decrease sun sensitivity, and

help care for skin during and after radiation therapy.

Relieve itching

This is a list of ideas for what you can do on your own to relieve itching.

➤ **Suggest bathing with cool water and using gentle soap.** Hot water can damage and dry out skin tissues. Harsh soaps are also too drying and should be avoided. Try an oatmeal soap or one with oil. Alpha Keri™ may be added to bath water. It eliminates the need for soap and softens the skin.

➤ **Add baking soda to bath water.** Baking soda soothes sensitive skin, decreases itching, and decreases the side effects of substances that naturally come out of the skin pores.

➤ **Remind the person with cancer to rinse skin thoroughly and pat dry.**

➤ **Apply cool, moist compresses to itchy areas.** Cool soaks are soothing and relieve itching at least for a short time. Use washcloths or soft dish towels soaked in cool water and wrung out.

➤ **Suggest keeping nails short and clean.** Shorter, well-filed nails are harder and less likely to scratch open the skin.

➤ **Encourage wearing clean white gloves, if scratching.** Clean white gloves over the hands help prevent scratching the skin with the nails. They are especially helpful at night when the person does not know that he or she is scratching.

➤ **Change bed sheets daily.** Dry skin flakes off and gathers on bed sheets. This can cause more itchiness and can further dry out the skin. Changing the sheets frequently removes the dry skin flakes and helps eliminate a buildup of bacteria. Fresh sheets bring a sense of comfort as well.

➤ **Wash sheets and towels in gentle laundry soap,** such as Dreft™ or Ivory Snow™. Harsh detergents remain on clothes, towels, and sheets and can cause itching and irritation.

➤ **Avoid harsh laundry detergents.** Detergents that attack oil or stains have more chemicals that are irritating to tender skin. Gentle detergents are made for softer, tender skin and should be used if skin problems occur.

➤ **Keep the room cool at 65 to 75 °F.** When the body sweats more, itchiness increases.

➤ **Encourage rest.** Too much activity makes the skin sweat. Rest cools the skin down again and decreases itchiness or skin irritation.

➤ **Avoid extreme cold or heat.**

➤ **Suggest covering up in the sun.** Heat from the sun causes sweating. Covering up also prevents sunburn and drying out of the skin. Use a lotion with at least a #15 sunblock.

Prevent dryness and itching

Dryness leads to itching. It can break the skin tissues to the point of cracking open. Here are a number of things you can encourage the person with cancer to do to prevent or treat dry skin:

➤ **Add mineral oil or baby oil to bath water.** The oil soaks in and prevents the water from drying out the skin.

➤ **Encourage taking sponge baths.** They are cooler and decrease the amount of time that the skin is immersed in water.

➤ **Avoid full baths or showers.** Taking a full bath or shower exposes all of your skin to heat for a longer time. This leads to increased dryness.

➤ **Use warm, not hot water.** Hot showers and tub baths expose more skin to drying heat.

➤ **Do not scrub the skin.** Scrubbing pulls on delicate skin tissues and removes important moisture.

➤ **Pat skin dry.** Patting is more gentle than rubbing and helps lock in needed moisture.

➤ **Suggest applying a mild, water-based moisturizing cream to skin when it is still slightly moist after a bath.** Water-based lotions replace needed moisture. Alcohol-based lotions actually can dry out the skin and should be avoided.

➤ **Limit bathing to once a day.** Bathing more than once a day leads to excessive dryness because the skin is rubbed and exposed to soap and hot water.

➤ **Encourage drinking 2 quarts of fluid every day, unless otherwise instructed.** Drinking fluids reduces the risk of dehydration and restores moisture to skin tissues.

➤ **Avoid extreme heat, cold, or wind.** Heat, cold, and wind chafe the skin, damaging it as well as drying it out.

➤ **Avoid colognes, after-shaves, or after-bath splashes that contain alcohol.** These also dry the skin.

➤ **Remind the person with cancer to use an electric razor.** Electric razors are less likely than razor blades to scrape off layers of skin.

➤ **Avoid opening or popping blisters.**

➤ **Put dry clean gauze on any open areas.**

Conceal dark skin, veins, or discolored fingernails

Skin pigment is affected by chemotherapy and often turns darker. <u>If this is troublesome to the person with cancer, suggest the following</u>:

➤ **Wear long sleeves to hide dark veins.** They also provide some protection against bumping or bruising.

➤ **Women may want to wear nail polish or a thin layer of make-up foundation.** Women can hide discolored nails with polish.

➤ **Keep nails clean, short, and filed smoothly.** Shorter nails show newer nail growth and are less likely to show deep discoloration.

Treat acne

Changes in skin pores and skin discharges can lead to blemishes that are both uncomfortable and unsightly. <u>Here are three things to do to prevent or treat acne</u>:

➤ **Keep skin clean with mild soap and warm water.** Harsh soaps inflame blemishes and strip the skin of important moisture.

➤ **Pat skin dry.** Gentle drying allows new skin to heal and doesn't irritate reddened or swollen areas.

➤ **Avoid astringents.** Although they dry out blemishes, astringents also dry the whole face and remove too much moisture. Keeping the skin clean is the best treatment for acne caused by chemotherapy.

Limit sweating

Chemotherapy can cause excessive amounts of perspiration. <u>You can help the person with cancer deal with this side effect in a variety of ways</u>.

➤ **Dress in two light layers of clothing.** The layer closest to the body should be cotton to absorb moisture. The outer layer should be light to allow air to pass through.

➤ **Change wet clothing as soon as possible.** Wet clothes lock in sweat, which can lead to chills and discomfort.

➤ **Avoid using cornstarch to absorb sweat.** When the white blood cell counts are low (which often happens after chemotherapy), do not use cornstarch because it can cause a skin fungus or yeast infection to develop. If you are uncertain about this, ask the nurse or doctor.

Decrease sun sensitivity

<u>Chemotherapy makes the skin tissue especially sensitive to the sun's rays, and sunburn occurs rapidly</u>.

➤ **Cover legs and arms.** Clothing stops the sun's rays from damaging the skin.

➤ **Wear lightweight fabrics.** They allow more air to pass through to the skin and keep it dry. Any covering also protects the skin from the sun's rays.

➤ **Wear a wide-brimmed hat and sunglasses.**

➤ **Use a suntan lotion with a sunblock of #15 or higher.** It prevents harmful rays from burning the skin.

➤ **Apply sunscreen to any newly exposed scalp.**

➤ **Stay in the sun only for a short time.**

➤ **Stay out of the sun from 11:00 am to 3:00 pm.** The sun is hottest and most dangerous during these hours. The skin tissues are very sensitive to these rays while the person with cancer is receiving certain chemotherapy drugs. Ask the doctor or nurse about this. They'll tell you if the drugs cause extra sensitivity to the sun.

➤ **Cover all skin appropriately when outdoors.** Be sure that arms and legs are totally covered if working outdoors. Use sunblock #15 on hands, face, and neck. Remind the person to re-apply sunblock at least every hour if hot and sweaty. Sunburn can occur in as short a time as 15 minutes of direct sunlight. He or she should also follow these tips on overcast days because ultraviolet rays can penetrate the clouds.

Take care of skin during and after radiation therapy

➤ **Wash with lukewarm water and mild soap.** Wash the skin gently and avoid hot or cold water. Do not scrub the skin because this irritates it. Lukewarm water and gentle rinsing is best.

➤ **Keep the treatment area clean and dry.** A daily sponge bath or lukewarm shower is recommended. If sweating occurs, cleanse afterwards.

➤ **Avoid using scented or medicated lotions, rubbing alcohol, creams, body oils, talcums, perfumes, and antiperspirants.** All of these skin ointments irritate the skin. Many leave a coating on the skin that can interfere with radiation therapy or healing. A special cream may be allowed by the radiation therapy department, but staff will recommend it and explain how to use it.

➤ **Avoid cornstarch to control perspiration.** Cornstarch will clump and cause a wet covering. Dusting with cornstarch or any talcum is to be avoided.

➤ **Avoid cornstarch in areas that are moist or wet.** Report wet skin areas to clinic staff, who will suggest how to treat them if they are near areas treated by radiation. Wet or moist areas are more likely to appear in skin folds, under the arms, and in the groin.

➤ **Avoid ice packs.** Ice irritates the skin. It constricts the blood vessels, which may inhibit healing.

➤ **Avoid hot water bottles and heating pads.** Heat can also irritate the skin.

➤ **Avoid direct sunlight to treated skin.** The ultraviolet rays of the sun can burn the treated skin easily because its skin cover is very tender during and after radiation. Avoid the sun for at least 1 year after radiation treatment.

➤ **Wear loose clothing.** Tight clothing causes redness and irritation. Loose clothing lets the skin breathe and does not restrict its flexibility.

➤ **Avoid scratching treated skin.** Scratching, rubbing, or scrubbing must be avoided. This can cause infection, irritation, or soreness. If itchiness is a problem, consult with the doctor or nurse.

Possible Obstacles

Think about what could stop you from carrying out your plan and how you would deal with it.

Here are three obstacles that other people have faced

1. "It's only the skin and not the body."

   Response: <u>Skin problems need to be treated early to prevent infection and to decrease discomfort</u>. If you notice changes, talk them over with the nurse or doctor. Don't wait until an infection or severe discomfort occurs.

2. "No one seems to know what to do about this itching. I guess we'll just have to live with it."

   Response: Itching is a difficult problem to heal. Try a combination of strategies to relieve constant itching. <u>Keep experimenting and visit a dermatologist, if necessary</u>.

3. "I'm afraid my skin will be fried by radiation therapy."

   Response: Radiation therapy does cause skin changes. The intention is not to "fry" the skin. Although it does get red and sensitive, the skin will heal. <u>Be sure to call for help, especially if the skin gets moist or wet and becomes sore</u>. Clinic staff keep a close watch on the skin, and the radiation therapist can stop the treatment and give the skin a rest.

Think of *other* obstacles that could interfere with carrying out your plan

What additional road blocks could get in the way of doing the things recommended in this home care plan? For example, will the person with cancer cooperate? Will other people help? How will you explain your needs to medical staff? Do you have the time and energy to carry out the plan?

You need to develop plans for getting around these road blocks. Use the four COPE ideas (creativity, optimism, planning, and expert information) in developing your plans. See the chapter on Solving Home Care Problems at the beginning of the book for a discussion of how to use the four COPE ideas in overcoming your obstacles.

Carrying Out and Adjusting Your Plan

Checking on results

Check the skin regularly to see if it has changed since radiation or chemotherapy began. Keep records of the skin problems that the person with cancer is having and of what helps or makes them worse.

If your plan doesn't work

If skin problems are getting worse, or if the person with cancer is becoming more and more uncomfortable or upset about these problems, review the section on What You Can Do To Help. If you have done all you can, then ask the nurse or doctor for help. Tell them what you have done and what the results have been.

Hair Loss

Overview of the
Home Care Plan for Hair Loss

Understanding the Problem

When to expect hair loss

What to expect when hair grows back

Questions to ask about hair loss

What You Can Do To Help

Caring for the scalp and coping with hair loss

Getting a wig or head cover

Possible Obstacles

"I can't afford a wig."

"I'll just have to live with it."

Carrying Out and Adjusting Your Plan

Plan in advance to find and use a wig

Ask a nurse, social worker, or hairstylist for help

(Topics with an arrow in front of them are actions you can take or symptoms you can look for.)

Hair Loss

[The information in this home care plan fits most situations, but yours may be different.

If the doctor or nurse tells you to do something else, follow what they say.]

Understanding the Problem

Some chemotherapy treatments can cause partial or complete hair loss. This may start as early as 7 to 14 days after treatment begins, and hair may not grow back until 6 to 12 months after chemotherapy treatments are completed. Radiation to the head causes permanent hair loss. Depending on where the radiation is directed, hair can also be lost on the eyelashes, eyebrows, pubic area, arms, underarms, chest, and legs. Usually, early hair growth is very fine, and the new hair may have a different texture. For example, if it was curly, it might come back straight. New hair may also be a different color because of a temporary absence of pigment in the hair shaft. If hair was brown, it might be lighter. Changes in color and texture are usually not permanent. Everyone's experience seems to be different.

Ask the physician, nurse, or technician what to expect about hair loss with the treatments that the person with cancer is receiving.

When will the hair loss start?

Will it fall out suddenly or slowly?

How much of the hair will be lost?

When will it grow back?

Your goals are to:

help the person with cancer delay or limit the amount of lost hair, and

live a normal life during the time that the hair is lost.

What You Can Do To Help

There are two things you can do to deal with this problem:

care for the scalp and cope with hair loss, and

get a wig or head cover.

Caring for the scalp and coping with hair loss

Chemotherapy weakens hair follicles, which causes hair to fall out quickly. Radiation to the head or scalp causes permanent hair loss to that area. At this point, <u>caring for the scalp is important to decrease itchiness and dryness</u>.

➤ **Brush and wash away hair that is falling out.**

➤ **Gently clean hair and scalp with a mild protein shampoo twice a week.** Use gentle shampoos for dry or damaged hair. These are mild and do not coat the hair with additional chemicals. Also massage the scalp to remove skin scales.

➤ **Use a protein conditioner.** Conditioners add body to fine or limp hair. It takes time for the new hair shafts to become thick.

➤ **Avoid hair care products that contain bleach, peroxide, ammonia, alcohol, or lacquer.** Avoid harsh chemicals. Select hair-styling products such as mousses, sprays, or gels that have light or normal hold. These can be shampooed out. Stronger products build up on hair shafts and can damage remaining hair or new hair.

➤ **Avoid heat, curling irons, hot rollers, or blow dryers as much as possible.** Gently dry hair with a blow dryer set at the lowest setting. Keep the heat farther away from the scalp than usual because the skin is sensitive and may easily burn.

➤ **Keep hair short and easy to style.** New hair breaks easily. Long hair requires more curling, pinning, and combing than short hair. Keeping hair easy to style decreases the amount of combing or styling of delicate hair.

➤ **Avoid braids or ponytails and use a wide-toothed comb.** Pulling breaks very fragile hair. Comb it gently with a wide-toothed comb.

➤ **Consider perming thin hair during chemotherapy.** During the chemotherapy cycle when only part of the hair has been lost, perming thin hair makes it look fuller. The perm won't damage the remaining hair. Do not use a home perm kit, though. Check with a hairstylist who will help decide when it is safe to perm.

➤ **Postpone a perm on *new* hair until after three haircuts or trims.** After chemotherapy, let new hair grow in and wait until the hair is at least 3 inches long to get a very mild body wave that lasts for a short time. Permanent waves cannot be tolerated by the scalp until at least 9 months after chemotherapy.

➤ **Protect the head and newly exposed skin from the sun with a hat and sunblock of #15 or higher.** Sun rays also dry the scalp and can burn it more readily than usual.

➤**Use a satin pillow or hair net while sleeping.** A satin pillow prevents tangling, and hair sheds more evenly when held in a net.

➤**Wear a hat or a head scarf to hold in heat in cold weather.** Because heat is lost through the top of the head, keeping the head warm retains body heat and protects the scalp from drying out in colder, harsh weather.

➤**Wear sunglasses to protect the eyelashes.** Even eyelashes are sensitive to chemotherapy and can be easily broken. Protection from the sun and cold weather is recommended.

➤**Men should gently wash off loose hair from the chest, face, pubic area, arms, underarms, and legs.**

➤**Women should gently wash off loose hair from the pubic area, arms, underarms, and legs.**

Getting a wig or head cover

➤**Ask a hairstylist about buying a wig.** Hairstylists can call a wig supplier and order catalogs. They can describe the different kinds of wigs to the person with cancer and order the wig. Many stylists have done this before, and many are willing to go to your home if you ask them.

➤**Call a wig shop in the phone book, and talk with professionals early about wigs.** If you plan to buy a wig, be prepared to pay $30 or more. Some wigs cost as much as $100. Major department stores carry wigs, if there is no specialty wig shop near you. Many people prefer to have their hairstylist order and style a wig that's just right.

➤**Match a small lock of the person's hair with a wig color before starting chemotherapy.** Wigs come in many colors and textures. A close match can be made between the person's hair and the wig piece. You might even want to try a new color. Again, a hairstylist is the best consultant on this.

➤**Ask about borrowing a wig, if you can't buy one.** Most offices of the American Cancer Society can tell you how to obtain or borrow a wig. Many of them have a "Wig Bank" with different types of wigs that they can loan or give. If their office staff reports that they don't have a Wig Bank, ask them to refer you to another American Cancer Society office that does. This second office can send wigs to them, and a Cancer Society volunteer can bring them to the home.

➤**Take the wig to a hairstylist to be styled.** Do this before all the hair is lost, and have the wig styled similar to the hairstyle before chemotherapy. When you get a wig, take it to a hairstylist who will help design it and style it for the best appearance. They can even cut it if it's too big or heavy. They will teach you how to care for it so that it keeps looking nice.

➤**Practice wearing the wig at home.** The person will be more comfortable in public after wearing the wig at home and learning how to bend over with it on.

➤**Return the wig to the hairstylist for repair or resetting.** Sometimes the hairpiece needs to be refreshed or restyled just the way normal hair does. Hairstylists know how to do this and can do it at a regular appointment. They can also cut the real hair, advise on scalp treatments, and give support and advice about the problems of hair loss.

➤**Try turbans, scarfs, hats, or caps.** Many stores sell attractive terry cloth or cotton turbans. Some hospital gift shops carry these also. Head coverings protect against drafts, enhance appearance, and retain body heat.

➤**Talk with other people who have lost their hair because of cancer treatments about what they did and how they coped.** Different people cope differently with this problem. Some accept baldness and do not cover their heads except in cold weather. Others feel that wigs or turbans are important and helpful. Getting their ideas helps the person with cancer judge what will be best for him or her.

Possible Obstacles

Think about what ideas or attitudes could stop you from carrying out this plan.

Here are some obstacles that other people have faced, which prevented them from trying to solve a problem with hair loss

1. "I can't afford a wig."

   Response: <u>Some insurance companies (basic coverage or major medical) cover part or all of the cost of wigs because it is needed after a medical problem</u> and is not for purely cosmetic reasons. To get insurance coverage, you might need a prescription. Have the physician write "wig for alopecia" or "full cranial prosthesis" on the prescription.

The cost of a wig can also be added to your medical expenses when doing income taxes. The American Cancer Society may help with the cost if they agree there is a financial need. <u>Nurses or social workers can help you get information about financial help and about insurance coverage</u>. In addition, local hairstylists may have free wig services. Ask what they offer to someone who can't afford to buy one.

2. "People say that he'll just have to live with being bald or having patches of hair on his head."

Response: Appearance can be very important to the person with cancer. Losing one's hair can be quite upsetting. Try not to expect your friend or family member to react the way you think you would to hair loss. Remember: <u>Helping a person look their best during a difficult time in their life can boost spirits and give confidence</u>.

Think of *other* obstacles that could interfere with carrying out your plan

What additional road blocks could get in the way of doing the things recommended in this home care plan? For example, will the person with cancer cooperate? Will other people help? How will you explain your needs to medical staff? Do you have the time and energy to carry out the plan?

You need to develop plans for getting around these road blocks. Use the four COPE ideas (creativity, optimism, planning, and expert information) in developing your plans. See the chapter on Solving Home Care Problems at the beginning of the book for a discussion of how to use the four COPE ideas in overcoming your obstacles.

Carrying Out and Adjusting Your Plan

Carrying out your plan

<u>If possible, decide in advance whether the person with cancer wants a wig</u> and what kind of a wig he or she wants. Order it as soon as possible. Meanwhile, follow the steps listed in this plan to slow down hair loss.

If your plan doesn't work

<u>If your plan does not seem to be working or hair loss is getting worse and you both feel badly about it, ask the social worker, nurse, or hairstylist for help</u>. Tell them what you have done and what the results have been.

Sexual Problems

Overview of the
Home Care Plan for Sexual Problems

Understanding the Problem

Sexual problems from cancer can have physical causes, emotional causes, or both

Ways to adjust to sexual changes due to cancer and cancer treatments

How cancer and cancer treatments can affect sexual functioning for women and men

Ostomies and sexual functioning

When To Get Professional Help

Symptoms and feelings that indicate that professional help is needed

Not all professionals will be knowledgeable about these issues—persist until your questions are answered

What You Can Do To Help

What women with cancer can do to improve sexual functioning and pleasure

What men with cancer can do to improve sexual functioning and pleasure

How to prevent infection from sexual contacts

Possible Obstacles

"Who would think of sex at a time like this?"

"She/he is concerned about sex, but doesn't want to talk about it."

"I am afraid to have intercourse or do anything like we used to do."

"Sex should be natural and spontaneous. If we have to work at it, it doesn't count."

"Men should be the ones to make sexual advances."

Carrying Out and Adjusting Your Plan

Sex is a sensitive subject for most people—think carefully about how you will discuss this subject with the person with cancer

Be patient and let the person with cancer move at a pace that is comfortable for him or her

If problems persist or are upsetting, get professional help, and persist until you get the help you need

(Topics with an arrow in front of them are actions you can take or symptoms you can look for.)

Sexual Problems

[The information in this home care plan fits most situations, but yours may be different.

If the doctor or nurse tells you to do something else, follow what they say.]

Understanding the Problem

Cancer and cancer treatments can affect a person's sexual behavior and pleasure, and adjusting to those changes is an important part of coping with the illness. To understand the changes that can occur, you should be aware of the four phases of the sexual response:

Desire is an interest in sex, with thoughts about it and feelings of attraction.

Excitement is when one feels aroused. Touching causes excitement, and the body responds by breathing faster, increasing the pulse and heart beat, and sending blood to the genital area. Men usually get erections when they are excited, and women's vaginas get wider and deeper.

Orgasm occurs when muscles contract around the genitals in rhythms that give intense pleasure. (Women's orgasms can come close together. Men may take more time between orgasms, especially as they get older.)

Resolution is the phase when one returns to an unexcited state. The heart beat decreases, and blood flows out of the genital area. Resolution usually happens within a few minutes after orgasm. If an orgasm does not occur, resolution takes longer.

Cancer and cancer treatments can affect any of these phases and often affect more than one. It is important for the person with cancer and his or her partner to understand why sexual changes are happening, to know what to expect, and to know what they can do to deal with or adjust to those changes.

Sexual problems from cancer can have physical causes, emotional causes, or both. Physically, very few cancer treatments injure parts of the body that give orgasms or sexual enjoyment. Exceptions include treatments that affect the brain or spinal cord, certain surgeries such as mastectomy (removal of a breast) or orchiectomy (removal of testicles), drugs that change normal hormone balance, and radiation therapy to the lower abdominal and genital areas. Intercourse or sexual touching may be impaired after these treatments, but people can still find feelings of pleasure. Side effects of treatments such as pain, nausea, or fatigue can also impair or reduce sexual pleasure. Finally, changes in the way a man or woman feels about their attractiveness can change responses in any of the four phases listed above.

Emotional obstacles to sexual pleasure and functioning include worry, which may distract one's attention from relaxing or from enjoying pleasure. Depression or anxiety can also prevent a person with cancer from feeling attractive or experiencing desire. It's important that people with cancer and their partners understand the reasons for changes in their desire to feel or give sexual pleasure. Sexual matters should be discussed with sensitivity to each other's feelings and with an openness to new ways of experiencing sexual closeness and pleasure.

Adjusting to sexual changes due to cancer and cancer treatments

➤ **Talk over feelings or concerns.** The person with cancer should discuss any fears or questions with his or her sexual partner. Talking about sexual matters with a close friend or medical professional can also help. Although many people find it difficult to talk about sexual matters, talking can help by clarifying what is important and what is of concern to each partner.

➤ **Plan periods of time for intimacy when you will not be interrupted.** Privacy is important for relaxation and sexual pleasure. Planning for uninterrupted time might be difficult, but it will help the person with cancer and the partner give the time and attention to intimacy that is needed.

➤ **A great deal of pleasure comes from touching and being held.** Sexual intimacy can be achieved without intercourse, without orgasms, and without erections or ejaculations. Being held and touched is an important part of all sexual intimacy and may be even more important when other sexual activities are restricted. Intimacy can be expressed by holding hands, putting an arm around the waist or shoulders, rubbing the back or arms and legs, and any other type of touching. Touch brings comfort and security.

Knowing that one is accepted and loved goes a long way to helping a person cope with cancer.

How cancer and cancer treatments can affect sexual functioning

Women

Most cancer treatments do not change a woman's basic ability to enjoy sexual feelings. However, some treatments do change or remove a woman's sexual organs or body parts, in which case problems may occur with resuming intercourse, with female genitals becoming lubricated or "wet" before intercourse, or with the woman's ability to reach orgasm. For example, after a vulvectomy, orgasm is no longer possible because the clitoris is removed. Other surgeries may affect pleasure. If the vagina is shortened because of cancer surgery, a woman may find that she cannot enjoy former positions during foreplay or intercourse and activities that used to bring pleasure. She will need to try new positions with her partner. She also may need to add moisture to her vagina if vaginal dryness becomes a problem. Female hormone levels may be affected by cancer or cancer treatments, which will also affect sexual interest. Worries and emotional problems can also affect a woman's sexual interest and responsiveness.

Breast surgery can affect a woman's feelings about her sexuality. If a breast is removed, the woman may feel differently about her sexual attractiveness. Adjusting to this physical change takes different lengths of time, depending on the woman's age, security in her sexual relationships, and the degree to which physical appearance is important to her.

Men

For men, most cancers or cancer treatments do not change how they respond to sexual stimulation or contact. However, some treatments (such as radiation to the pelvis and some chemotherapies or surgeries) do change a man's sexual response. Erections can become difficult or impossible, ejaculation may stop, or orgasms may diminish in frequency or intensity. Psychological changes, mood changes, and worries can also make a difference in men's responses to sexual situations.

One reason for decreased desire or sexual function in a man is damage or injury to blood vessels and nerves in the pelvic area. Blood vessels and nerves stimulate the penis, scrotum, and surrounding area to feel aroused, gain an erection, produce sperm, and ejaculate sperm. Damage to the nerves or blockage to the blood vessels from cancer or cancer treatments can prevent erections or make semen production impossible. In spite of this, many of these men can still feel aroused, feel pleasure, and reach orgasm. Many can even ejaculate with or without an erection, and many can feel an orgasm (or "climax") without ejaculating sperm. This is known as "dry orgasm" and is discussed in more detail later in this home care plan.

Some cancer or cancer treatments can affect testosterone (male hormone) levels. Low levels of testosterone, which is produced by the testicles and adrenal glands, can cause trouble with erections or feelings of sexual desire and may decrease the intensity of the orgasm. Nerve damage can also diminish pleasure and increase discomfort. For example, nerve damage at the prostate gland, or where the urine pours out, can cause pain during ejaculation.

Radiation therapy can also change the ability to have and keep an erection, depending on how much radiation is given and how much of the pelvis is exposed to it. The more radiation and the wider the area of skin exposed, the more likely are problems with erections. For example, radiation therapy can injure arteries in the penis, which can result in less blood flow into the penis for creating or keeping an erection. Chemotherapy can also decrease desire and the ability to have erections, and some cancer medications can reduce testosterone levels and create hormonal imbalances. Hormone levels usually return to normal after cancer chemotherapy ends, and the effects of radiation and chemotherapy are often temporary. But damage to nerves and organs from surgery remains. Adjusting to these changes is part of learning to live with a diagnosis of cancer.

Ostomies and sexual functioning

Some cancer surgeries result in the person with cancer having an ostomy. An ostomy is a surgical opening in the skin to pass stool, urine, or both. The stool or urine is usually collected in a bag that is worn outside the skin. A person's sexual behaviors and feelings about sex are often affected by having an ostomy.

Nurses and surgeons who care for people with ostomies are familiar with the kinds of problems people have adjusting to this operation and can usually give advice for sexual adjustments, too. Enterostomal therapists are nurses who specialize in helping people learn how to manage their ostomies. They can give advice and information to help ostomy patients adjust sexually.

People with ostomies often find help with their problems, including sexual ones, from an ostomy club, where groups of people get together to talk about living with an ostomy. Club members gather to share information, teach, and support each other. They meet monthly or every other month and usually issue a small newsletter. Meeting with them gives the person with cancer a chance to talk with other people and families who have learned to live with a colostomy, urinary ostomy, or both. They can help you learn about new products and ways to manage the ostomies and skin around them and can also discuss concerns such as controlling odors or making sexual contact.

Your goals are to:

be fully informed about the sexual effects of cancer and cancer treatments and what can be done to deal with these effects,

to prevent infections from sexual contacts, and

to help the person with cancer experience as much sexual closeness and pleasure as he or she desires.

When To Get Professional Help

You should talk to the doctor or nurse if the person with cancer is experiencing any of the following

➤ **Pain during intercourse.** Any pain with intercourse is a reason to talk to a doctor. Women should report painful intercourse to her gynecologist and ask for advice about trying other positions or about continuing intercourse. If a gynecologist has not been involved, report this pain to the surgeon or doctor in charge, who can advise her on whom to turn to for help or further examination.

Men should also report pain with intercourse and any redness on or unusual discharge from the penis.

Radiation therapy to the abdominal or pelvic area may also cause pain during intercourse for both men and women. If this happens, it should be reported and discussed with the radiation oncologist.

➤ **Questions about when to have intercourse.** Sometimes people are reluctant to talk about their sexual activities. However, it is best to be open and to ask the doctor or nurse about when to resume intercourse. It is also important to ask about symptoms that may be a sign to stop intercourse.

➤ **A sexual partner who is fearful.** Some partners may want to resume sexual activity but are afraid because they fear they will hurt the person with cancer, spread the cancer, or even get cancer themselves. Both the partner and the person with cancer should talk over these concerns with doctors and nurses. They will be told that cancer is not contagious and that it will not spread because of sexual activity. They can also ask questions about pain and may be given suggestions about new positions or sexual and touching practices.

➤ **Concern because of having little or no interest in sexual activities or feelings.** If the person with cancer or the partner is concerned about having little interest in sexual intercourse, they should discuss the problem with a doctor or nurse who can explain the causes and when sexual interest may be expected to return.

> **Inability or unwillingness to talk about changes in sexual activities or feelings, even when asked.** Talking about sexual issues can be difficult, especially if the person with cancer has not talked openly about sex in the past, feels unattractive, or does not want to admit to having sexual problems.

Note that not all professionals will be knowledgeable about these issues. Therefore, if the first professional you talk to can't help, keep looking. Ask for a referral to a professional who has experience helping people with these problems.

What You Can Do To Help

Women with cancer

Treatments and surgery in the pelvic or abdominal area can change sexual responses or a woman's willingness to touch intimately. For example, women who have had hysterectomies, urinary surgery, or surgery that increases the likelihood of urine leaking can benefit from these suggestions.

> **Empty the bladder before intercourse or before touching.** Muscles around the opening to the vagina may have been weakened by surgery. The opening to the tube that carries urine out of the body may also have been weakened. Emptying the bladder before sexual touching or intercourse decreases the chance of urine leaking out. In addition, pressure from urine in the bladder can impair relaxation because the woman is concerned that urine may leak. Also, the urinary pressure may be more noticeable than any feelings of pleasure.

If the woman is catheterizing herself to drain urine, empty the bladder before any type of sexual activity. Some women, whose urinary system has been injured after surgery or because of cancer, may need to catheterize themselves every few hours to remove urine from the bladder. They may have to do this for a short time or permanently. In either case, it is wise to self-catheterize before any sexual activity. Again, feelings of fullness in the bladder can interfere with feelings of sexual relaxation and pleasure.

> **Lubricate the vagina with a water-based gel before sexual activity.** Some cancer treatments make the vagina drier and take longer to make fluids that aid intercourse. Vaginal dryness can also happen because of aging or general worry about having sex. Dryness can be caused by medicines, including some chemotherapies, by radiation treatment, and by surgery. Dryness can be treated by lubricating the vagina with a water-based gel before

sexual activity. Water-based gels can be spread inside the vagina and also outside on the skin around the vaginal opening. Gels come in tubes or jars, or as suppositories, which melt in the vagina. Some brands can be used a few times during the week to help soften and moisturize the vagina and outside skin; these brands do not have to be used every day or before every intercourse. Vaginal gels that are water-based can be bought at drugstores or pharmacies without a prescription. For best results, look for a gel that does *not* have an alcohol base but, instead, is water-based.

➤ **If the person with cancer is taking hormones for cancer, learn what changes to expect in sexual feelings and responses and how long these changes will last.** Sometimes, anti-estrogens are prescribed to reduce the risk of getting breast cancer again, but they may have side effects such as shakiness or hot flashes. Find out when side effects will appear, how long they will last, and when they will disappear. Also, ask how anti-estrogens may affect vaginal wetness or feelings of desire and excitement. The doctor or nurse can tell you what these drugs do and what side effects to expect.

➤ **If the person with cancer is receiving chemotherapy or radiotherapy, learn what changes to expect in sexual feelings and responses and how long these changes will last.** Some chemotherapy medicines and radiotherapy treatments cause changes in vaginal wetness and in normal sexual responses. Ask the nurse or doctor about this. Pharmacists may also be able to help you find this information.

➤ **If the person with cancer has had a mastectomy, lumpectomy, or post-mastectomy reconstruction for breast cancer, call the American Cancer Society and ask a Reach to Recovery volunteer to visit.** Your local American Cancer Society will assign a volunteer who has had breast cancer, surgery, and treatment. These volunteers visit the person with cancer in the hospital and at home. They demonstrate arm exercises to do after surgery, explain what to expect in healing and using the arm on the surgical side, and discuss dressing, bras, and breast prostheses. They can also answer questions about sexuality, feeling attractive, and sexual activities.

Cancer Society volunteers can also discuss what to expect after a lumpectomy and the pros and cons of breast reconstruction after mastectomy. The Cancer Society will send a volunteer who is closely matched to the person she is visiting so that they can share experiences and talk about problems recovering and resuming everyday activities.

➤**Find out if the cancer treatments cause infertility (not being able to have a child).** Some cancer surgeries or treatments result in female infertility. For example, when the ovaries or uterus are removed, a woman can no longer have a child. High-dose radiation may also result in infertility. If the person with cancer becomes infertile, there are other ways to have children, such as through adoption or having another woman carry the child.

Men with cancer

➤**Ask if "dry" orgasms will happen.** Certain surgeries and treatments cause more sex-related nerve and blood vessel damage than others. Nerve and blood vessel injury near the penis or prostate, or in the pelvic area, changes the way men experience desire, erections, and orgasms. They can also affect whether they continue to ejaculate. Sometimes they ejaculate into the bladder because muscles and openings have changed or weakened after surgery. In this case, urine is cloudy because it is mixed with seminal fluid and sperm.

When a man has the feeling of an orgasm, but no ejaculation comes out, it is called a "dry orgasm." Women do not notice a difference during lovemaking. Men can still have erections and enjoy sexual pleasure without the wet sperm ejaculation that they knew in the past. However, it will take time to adjust to this change.

➤**If the person with cancer might want to father children in the future, find out if banking sperm is an option.** Some cancer surgeries and treatments, such as removal of the testicles or high-dose radiation therapy, especially in the genital area, result in sterility. This means that a man is no longer able to make a baby. If you or the person with cancer are concerned about sterility, ask the doctor about banking sperm, especially if there is even the slight possibility that he may want to be a future father. Sperm is collected by the man before the surgery or treatment and frozen (or "banked") for future use, when it can be planted through artificial insemination in a woman's womb to make her pregnant.

➤**If the person with cancer is taking hormone drugs as a cancer treatment, learn what changes to expect and how long they will last.** Sometimes, the level of testosterone falls after cancer surgery or treatments. A low testosterone level can cause problems with erections and even lower sexual desire. Your doctor can check testosterone blood levels, and, if they are too low, additional testosterone drug doses can be ordered. However, in the case of prostate cancer, male hormones are not given because they can speed up the growth of prostate cancer.

Another hormone commonly given is DES or diethylstilbesterol. If the person with cancer is taking this hormone, be sure that you and he know about its expected side effects and when they will appear, including how DES may change sexual responses such as erections or feelings of desire.

➤ **If erections may be a problem after treatment or surgery, ask about penis implants (also called penile implants).** If the man with cancer wants to have more success with erections, penile implants or prostheses are an option. Some create a permanent or semirigid erection that can be hidden under clothes. Other implants are inflatable, which gives a man more control over when to have an erection. In this case, a small pump is placed under the skin, and the erection occurs because the man pushes the pump several times, usually to let water fill tubes placed inside the penis. Other types of implants are also available. Surgeons and urologists know about the options and can discuss the pros and cons of each with the person with cancer and his sexual partner.

Prevent infection from sexual contacts

Infections can happen from sexual contacts when the immune system is functioning poorly as a result of chemotherapy or radiotherapy treatments. Here are some things that can be done to prevent infections:

➤ **Urinate after sex.** Urinating after sex rinses out bacteria that may cause infection. After sexual activity, new bacteria are left near the urinary tract. Should the immune system be impaired, these bacteria can lead to an infection, not just in the urinary tract, but elsewhere, too. Ask the doctor about whether the person with cancer risks infection more than usual by having sexual contact.

➤ **Wash hands before and after sexual contact and after using the bathroom.** Thorough hand washing is the most important way to prevent infection caused by touching the genitals and caressing.

➤ **Avoid sexual contact with people who may have infectious and transmissible diseases like colds, flu, or cold sores.** This includes all infectious diseases, from colds to sexually transmitted diseases, including AIDS. Condoms can help prevent the spread of infectious diseases, but they are not 100% effective for all infections.

➤ **Clean the rectum thoroughly after bowel movements.** Infections are easily spread from bacteria around the anus to the opening of the vagina or penis. The best way to prevent this is to gently wash the anus and surrounding skin with warm water and soap.

Possible Obstacles

Here are obstacles that other people have faced in dealing with sexual problems from cancer

1. "Who would think of sex at a time like this?"

   Response: Sexual feelings and thoughts can happen anytime, and it is normal to have them. They may be caused by a need for being close and for being held, for feeling loved, secure, and accepted. Sexual activities may also distract a person from worries.

2. "He (she) is concerned about sex, but doesn't want to talk about it."

   Response: You can mention to the doctor or nurse that he or she is concerned about sex, and they can raise the issue when talking with him or her. You can also ask about whether a "sex therapist" works in your area. These professionals specialize in helping people learn or re-learn how to enjoy sexual contact. Often their fees are covered by insurance if your visits are ordered by a doctor. Often only a few visits are needed to give you ideas about what to do and how to cope with changes in sexual life.

3. "I am afraid to have intercourse or do anything like we used to do."

   Response: It may take time to try new ways of touching or having intercourse. Use the booklets written by the American Cancer Society on sex and cancer. They are full of useful information on understanding changes in the body and also full of tips about ways to try new positions and get as well as give sexual pleasure. Talk with a trusted health care professional, too. He or she will understand your concerns and help you with ideas on how to give and receive sexual enjoyment.

   No matter how old a person is, being touched and held are important ways to show affection and feel comforted, even if you must postpone or give up intercourse.

4. "Sex should be natural and spontaneous. If we have to work at it, it doesn't count."

> Response: Some sexual behaviors, such as touching and holding, can always be spontaneous. Others, such as having a sexual climax, may require some planning and experimenting. Even then, they can still be enjoyed. Cancer changes many things, and sexual activity may be one of them. Having an open, flexible attitude will help you to have the most sexual pleasure possible under these new conditions.

5. "Men should be the ones to make sexual advances."

> Response: There is no law that says that only men should make sexual advances. Cancer can change many parts of a person's life, and the best way to adjust is to be flexible and to experiment with new ways of doing things.

Carrying Out and Adjusting Your Plan

Carrying out your plan

Sex is a sensitive subject for most people. Think carefully about what you will do and especially how you will discuss the subject with the person with cancer.

The section on Working and Communicating Effectively with the Person with Cancer in the home care plan for Succeeding at Caregiving has suggestions for how to discuss sensitive subjects and how to let the person with cancer know that you are available to talk when they are ready. Be patient and let the person with cancer move at a pace that is comfortable for him or her.

Health professionals can be very helpful. They are often skilled in raising and discussing sexual matters. However, not all professionals are skilled or knowledgeable. Therefore, if the first professionals you talk to are not helpful with sexual problems, persist until you find ones that are.

If your plan doesn't work

If sexual concerns remain a problem, your plan does not seem to be working, or these problems are happening more often, re-read the section on When To Get Professional Help in this home care plan. If any of the conditions listed there exist, call the doctor or nurse for advice and a referral to someone you can talk with.

Recommended Reading

The American Cancer Society distributes two excellent pamphlets: *Sexuality and Cancer: For the Woman Who Has Cancer and Her Partner* and *Sexuality and Cancer: For the Man Who Has Cancer and His Partner*. Both of these pamphlets are available without charge from your local American Cancer Society unit.

Maintaining Positive Experiences

Overview of the
Home Care Plan for Maintaining Positive Experiences

Understanding the Problem

Why it is important to keep up positive experiences during an illness

How this protects against depression

People caring for someone with cancer should keep up positive experiences, too

When To Get Professional Help

If the person with cancer feels it is impossible to have positive experiences, read the home care plan for Coping with Depression for guidance about when to get professional help

What You Can Do To Help

Three types of positive experiences

How to pay more attention to positive experiences

How to arrange and organize positive experiences

A place to list pleasant, involving activities that the person with cancer can do now

Possible Obstacles

"Nothing is pleasant anymore."

"You can't do anything about the bad things that happen when you're sick."

"There are too many problems for the family caregiver to find time for pleasant activities."

The family caregiver feels guilty about doing enjoyable things when the person with cancer is sick.

Carrying Out and Adjusting Your Plan

Start now—don't wait until problems build up

Set deadlines to plan and have positive experiences

Be sure your goals are reasonable

Ask other people for suggestions

Examples of Positive Activities and Experiences

(Topics with an arrow in front of them are actions you can take or symptoms you can look for.)

Maintaining Positive Experiences

Understanding the Problem

People with cancer tend to focus their attention on their problems. As a result, they may withdraw from the people and activities they normally enjoy. For example, they may stop seeing friends or lose interest in a favorite hobby, and the quality of their lives may suffer.

Pleasant, satisfying experiences help people cope with cancer and other serious problems. Having fun makes people feel better physically and emotionally. When people regularly do things they enjoy, they keep a positive outlook on life and are less likely to become depressed during a difficult illness like cancer.

One of the most important things a caregiver can do for the person with cancer is to help that person find a balance between his or her problems and the enjoyable things in life.

Your goal is to arrange as many pleasant, positive experiences as possible for the person with cancer during this illness.

(Persons caring for someone with cancer can also become preoccupied with their problems. They should remember to do things they enjoy, too, in order to maintain a positive outlook. Caregivers who think only about the needs and problems of the person with cancer are likely to become upset and discouraged. As a result, they may no longer give their best care. Caregivers should read this plan for themselves as well as for the persons under their care.)

When To Get Professional Help

If the person with cancer feels that it is impossible for him or her to have any positive experiences, and, at the same time, is feeling sad and depressed, then professional help is needed.

Read the home care plan on Coping with Depression for guidance about when and how to get professional help for depression.

What You Can Do To Help

There are three types of positive experiences that are important in maintaining good quality of life and in helping prevent depression.

➤ **Enjoyable activities with other people:** doing things with people who like and respect you and whom you enjoy being with. Examples are:

Talking about sports with a friend

Shopping with a friend

Going to the beach with the family

Calling a friend on the phone

Being in a play

Going to a party

Playing cards with friends

Playing with grandchildren

Gossiping with friends

Going to church with family

Singing in a choir

Attending a fraternal organization or service club meeting

➤ **Important activities that give the person a sense of accomplishment:** activities that he or she feels are important and that give them a sense of pride. Examples are:

Cooking a fancy meal

Building a snowman

Repairing a broken lamp

Starting a new hobby

Jogging

Solving a crossword puzzle

Writing a letter

Volunteering to help needy people

Playing a musical instrument

Restoring old furniture

Cleaning the stove

Writing a poem

➤ **Activities that make the person feel good:** doing things or thinking about things that are especially pleasant and that lead to feelings that are the opposite of feeling depressed. Examples are:

Watching a favorite TV program

Watching a funny movie

Taking a ride in the country

Listening to a favorite kind of music

Reading a favorite magazine

Walking along the shore

Hugging someone you love

Eating a special food

Saying a prayer

Playing with a pet

Going to a religious service

Reading a joke book

There are two things you can do to ensure that the person with cancer has these three types of positive experiences.

1. You can help him or her pay attention to positive things that happen.
2. You can arrange and organize pleasant activities.

Pay attention to positive experiences

➤ **Talk about pleasant experiences as they happen during the day.** It is easy to notice and think just about unpleasant experiences when you are under stress. When this happens, it can make you and the person with cancer depressed. Make a point of noticing and talking about pleasant things as they happen; this helps to keep a balance between pleasant and unpleasant experiences.

➤ **Set aside a special time each evening when you and the person with cancer talk about the good things that happened that day.** Think back over the day and talk with the person with cancer about everything that was pleasant. Be sure to include all three categories: pleasant things that happened with other people, activities that gave a sense of pride and accomplishment, and activities that made him or her feel good.

➤ **Make lists of pleasant experiences.** This is helpful to many people because the pleasant experiences seem more definite or real when they see them written down.

Keep these lists and read them over from time to time to remind him or her about the good things in life. After you have done this for awhile, you both will find yourselves noticing good things as they happen and telling yourselves "I'll write that down tonight." And, best of all, you'll start the day looking forward to the positive things that will happen.

Arrange and organize pleasant activities

➤ **Make a list of activities that have been pleasant and enjoyable in the past.** You should do this with the person with cancer as well as with other family members and friends who have done pleasant activities with him or her. Be imaginative—think of as many activities as you can for each category. Include activities that have been pleasant during the illness as well as before the illness.

➤ **Decide what part of the activities the person with cancer can do now.** Some of the activities won't require any changes, but others may have to be changed because of limitations due to the illness. If you need to change an item, erase it and write what the person with cancer can do now in its place.

If the person with cancer can't do an activity, ask yourself:

a. Can he or she do some part of it?

b. Can he or she do something similar to that activity?

c. Can he or she talk about how to do that activity after the illness or treatments are over?

On the last page of this home care plan is a list of activities that other people have found enjoyable and rewarding. If you are having trouble remembering pleasant activities, this list may remind you.

The following is a form where you can list pleasant, enjoyable activities that the person with cancer can do now. We recommend that you fill in this form now and that you add to it throughout the illness. Then it will be ready to use whenever you need it.

Include all three types of pleasant activities:

enjoyable activities with other people,

activities that give a sense of pride and accomplishment, and

activities that make the person with cancer feel good.

A PLACE TO LIST PLEASANT, INVOLVING ACTIVITIES
THAT THE PERSON WITH CANCER CAN DO NOW

First, write activities for each category that the person with cancer has enjoyed in the past. Then write what part of those activities he or she can do now.

Enjoyable activities with other people

_____

_____

_____

_____

_____

_____

_____

Activities with a sense of accomplishment

_____

_____

_____

_____

_____

_____

_____

Activities that make him or her feel good

_____

_____

_____

_____

_____

_____

_____

_____

Here are examples of how past activities can be adjusted so that the person with cancer can do part of them or something like them now.

(Past activities are in light type and activities the person with cancer can do now are in **bold type**.)

Enjoyable activities with other people:

Shopping with friends — **Go through catalogs with Ann and Thelma**

Playing cards — **Invite Bill and Ann to play cards**

Dinner with John and Kay — **Invite John and Kay for dessert**

Watch grandson play baseball — **Watch baseball on TV with grandson**

Important activities that give a sense of accomplishment:

Cleaning basement — **Clean room**

Finishing jigsaw puzzle — **Start new puzzle**

Grass mowing — **Arrange to pay Billy to mow grass**

Sailing — **Build a model sailboat**

Activities that make him or her feel good:

Fred Astaire movies — **Rent video**

Cosby TV program — **Watch for reruns**

Dixieland jazz — **Play records after supper**

See grandchildren grow up — **Look through picture album**

See the last page of this home care plan for more examples of activities that other people have found enjoyable and rewarding.

Possible Obstacles

To make your plan work, you need to consider obstacles that could prevent you from carrying out your plan.

Here are some obstacles that people told us stood in their way in carrying out their plans to increase positive experiences

1. Person with cancer says, "No activity is pleasant anymore."

   Response: <u>No matter how depressed or upset someone is, there are always *some* activities and thoughts that are pleasant—even if it is only for a short time.</u> Start by noticing the good things that happen each day—even if they are small. Make lists of good things at the end of the day. Then try planning different activities until you find something that he or she responds to. It may be slow going at first but keep trying. You will often find that the person gradually becomes more and more responsive. <u>If the person with cancer is very depressed, he or she may need professional help</u>. Read the home care plan on Coping with Depression for ideas about what you can do to help control depression and about when to get professional help for depression.

2. "When you are sick, a lot of things happen that you wish wouldn't happen—but you can't do anything about them."

   Response: This home care plan will help you to balance your positive and negative experiences. <u>We can't do anything about many of the negative experiences due to an illness, but we can balance them with positive experiences</u>—that is what this care plan will help you to do.

3. "There are so many problems to deal with that the family caregiver can't find time for pleasant activities."

   Response: Family caregivers need to keep up pleasant activities as much as the person with cancer. <u>Pleasant activities are especially important for people who are under stress</u>! That is when they are needed the most. You need to make time for pleasant experiences, even in the midst of problems. If you just think about problems, you and the person with cancer will become sad and depressed.

4. The person caring for someone with cancer says, "I feel guilty if I enjoy myself when the person I'm caring for feels sick and needs my help."

   Response: You should be scheduling pleasant experiences for yourself as well as for the person you are caring for. You will be a better caregiver if you are in good spirits and doing things you enjoy. If you are depressed, you won't be able to do your best as a caregiver. Therefore, <u>scheduling pleasant experiences for yourself is part of being a good caregiver</u>.

Think of *other* obstacles that could interfere with carrying out your plan

What additional road blocks could get in the way of doing the things recommended in this home care plan? For example, will the person with cancer cooperate? Will other people help? How will you explain your needs to other people? Do you have the time and energy to carry out the plan?

You need to develop plans for getting around these road blocks. Use the four COPE ideas (creativity, optimism, planning, and expert information) in developing your plans. See the chapter on Solving Home Care Problems at the beginning of the book for a discussion of how to use the four COPE ideas in overcoming your obstacles.

Carrying Out and Adjusting Your Plan

Carrying out your plan

Start now

Don't wait until the person with cancer is depressed or feeling overwhelmed by problems. Start using this home care plan right away and then continue to use it throughout the illness. Start by noticing positive things as they happen. Then make lists of good things that happen at the end of the day, and, finally, schedule pleasant activities to do each week. Scheduling pleasant activities is one of the best ways to protect against depression.

Set deadlines

If you don't set deadlines to do these things, problems will push them aside. Therefore, you should decide, with the person with cancer, when you will do each of the activities you listed.

Checking on results

Your lists of good things that happen each day are a record of your progress. If the number or types of good things change, ask yourself why.

If the plan does not work

Don't be discouraged if you are not completely successful the first week. As you get more experience, you will get better and better at planning and noticing positive experiences. Ask yourself if your goals were reasonable. Perhaps you set goals that were too ambitious.

Ask other people to make suggestions for pleasant activities for the person who has cancer. Other experienced caregivers may have good ideas. Social workers and nurses who work with cancer patients often have good suggestions. Be creative. Try unusual and new ideas.

Examples of Positive Activities and Experiences

Examples of positive things that you can notice

<u>Enjoyable things that happened with other people</u>: Jerry said I looked good today; Martha went out of her way to get my medicine; the nurse was very understanding about how I felt; Tom did the dishes without complaining; Mary and I had a good talk; Bill and I talked about the old days.

<u>Activities that gave a sense of accomplishment</u>: I beat Charlie at chess; I stood up to the parking attendant and told him he was being rude; I finished knitting the arm to the sweater; I cleaned out my bureau drawers; I balanced the checkbook; I finished potting the flowers; I walked farther than I did yesterday.

<u>Activities that make me feel good</u>: I saw a bluebird; I enjoyed the shadows that the sun made coming through my window; I really laughed at the interview with the lobster fisherman on the evening news; I looked through our family album; I went to church; I ordered flowers for Ann, who is in the hospital; I encouraged Bill, who was just diagnosed with cancer.

Examples of pleasant activities you can plan

<u>Doing things with other people</u>: calling a friend on the phone, playing cards with friends, going to a party or social affair where there are people you like to be with, working on a project with a friend or family member.

<u>Doing important, rewarding activities</u>: working on a home improvement project, doing volunteer work, helping someone else.

<u>Doing things that make you feel happy</u>: watching a funny movie, hugging someone you love, watching people being happy, gardening, sports, walking, hobbies.

Getting Companionship and Support from Family and Friends

Overview of the Home Care Plan for
Getting Companionship and Support from Family and Friends

Understanding the Problem

Socializing with other people often drops off as the illness goes on

Some important kinds of support are lost when this happens

You should reach out to others to arrange as much socializing as the person with cancer needs and wants

Remember your own need for socializing

When To Get Professional Help

If the person with cancer is depressed about not having companionship, read the home care plan on Coping with Depression for guidance about when to get professional help

What You Can Do To Help

List people who can provide companionship

Plan how to make visiting pleasant for visitors

Don't wait for people to visit—seek them out

A place to write the names of people who can provide companionship and support

Possible Obstacles

"People should volunteer to visit without being asked."

"I'm afraid that I'll be turned down if I invite people or ask to visit them."

"Some people feel awkward talking to someone who is sick. They don't know what to say."

"The person I'm caring for doesn't want people to see him when he is sick."

"Some people are well meaning, but they boss us around or say things that are upsetting."

"Some people stay too long and tire us out."

Carrying Out and Adjusting Your Plan

Start with people who are easier to visit or invite, and then try people who are more challenging

If you are having problems carrying out your plan, ask other people to help you and give you ideas

Repeat these problem-solving steps regularly to ensure that the person with cancer has the companionship he or she wants and needs

(Topics with an arrow in front of them are actions you can take or symptoms you can look for.)

Getting Companionship and Support from Family and Friends

Understanding the Problem

When people are sick, it is normal for their families and friends to express interest and concern and to offer to help. While many people are interested and concerned early in the illness, often fewer and fewer people take the time and effort to visit or to call as the illness goes on. This happens for several reasons. People who are not sick are often uncomfortable around those who are, and so it is often easy to let other activities and problems become more important than visiting someone with an illness. Another reason is that some people with cancer withdraw from their friends and family, especially as their illness progresses. They do this because they don't want other people to see them when they are ill, they are not feeling well enough to make the effort, they don't want other people telling them what to do, or they feel that their friends should take the initiative to visit them. When friends and family see this withdrawal, they feel less welcome.

Unfortunately, <u>something important is lost when people with cancer see fewer and fewer people. They lose the stimulation of thinking about other people's lives, they lose the ability to see their own problems in a larger perspective, and they lose the suggestions and help which others can give. They also forget that other people love and care about them</u>.

<u>It is important that you, as a caregiver, do what you can to prevent social isolation</u>. You should invite people to visit, organize the visits so they are helpful to the person with cancer, and make the visit rewarding for the visitor so that he or she wants to come again. This home care plan will help you to do that.

Your goal is to:

arrange for as much social contact as the person with cancer needs and wants throughout the illness.

(Also remember that your own needs for companionship and support are important, too. You will be a better caregiver if you keep up your outside interests and relationships with other people during this illness. <u>You should use the ideas in this home care plan for yourself as well</u>. Planning time away with friends can be helpful. It can take your thoughts away from caregiving, and it can give you a chance to tell others about your feelings and experiences. It can also give others an opportunity to express their support to you and to make suggestions from their experiences.)

When To Get Professional Help

If the person with cancer feels that no one likes him or her, does not want to have companionship, and, at the same time, is feeling sad and depressed, then professional help is needed.

Read the home care plan on Coping with Depression for guidance about when and how to get professional help for depression.

What You Can Do To Help

There are three things you can do to make sure that the person with cancer gets the companionship and support he or she needs:

make a list of people who can provide companionship,

select people from this list and decide how you will make visiting pleasant for them, and

plan and arrange to visit them or for them to visit you.

<u>Don't wait for other people to ask to visit. Part of your job as a caregiver is to seek them out and to either visit them or invite them to visit you.</u>

Make a list of people who can provide companionship

➤**Make a list of companions.** <u>Make a list of the people who could give companionship and support to the person with cancer. Do this *with* the person you are caring for and with help from family members and friends. Try to make a long list</u>.

As you make your list, consider the following types of people:

Friends

Neighbors

Relatives

People who worked or went to school with the person with cancer

Members of the same community organizations such as churches, fraternal or community service organizations, political organizations, and so on

People with the same interests or hobbies

"Helpers"—people who have a lot of experience caring for sick people and are willing to give advice and help

➤ **Don't worry about how far away these people live, how busy they are, how long since you've talked to them, or even how well you know them.** If you are not sure whether to include someone, put them on the list. Your goal is to have the longest list you can. As you get experience with this home care plan, you will become more skilled and comfortable arranging for companionship, and, as that happens, you will want to contact more and more of the people on your list.

➤ **Telephone calls are often easier to arrange than inviting someone to the home.** If there are people to whom the person with cancer enjoys talking on the phone, be sure to include them on this list. You can encourage these people to call or you can make calls to them.

➤ **Helpers are often volunteers in community or church organizations,** or they may be friends or neighbors who have worked as nurses, teachers or counselors, or in social service agencies.

➤ **Pets are another kind of companion that have been helpful and supportive for many sick people.** If the person with cancer does not have a pet, he or she may want to consider getting one.

Decide how you will make visiting pleasant for them

On the next page of this home care plan is a form where you can list companions and note how to make visiting enjoyable for them. We recommend that you fill in this form now and that you add to it throughout the illness. Then it will be ready to use whenever you need it.

➤ **Thinking about the visit from the point of view of the other person will help you to make the visit more pleasant.** This will make you a better visitor and a better host or hostess and will also give you ideas for how to arrange visits, what to do when you are together, and how to increase the chances that you will get together again.

Next to each person on your list, write what he or she would like or enjoy about being with the person with cancer. Ask yourself, "What would make a visit really nice for him or her?"

➤ **The following are examples of how home caregivers have made visits enjoyable for their visitors.**

"Phil is a workaholic. That's all he thinks about. So when we get together, we ask him about work and he loves it."

A PLACE TO WRITE THE NAMES OF PEOPLE WHO CAN PROVIDE COMPANIONSHIP AND SUPPORT TO THE PERSON WITH CANCER

First, write the names of all the people who could give companionship and support. Make the longest list you can. Then, next to each name, write what he or she would enjoy doing when being with the person with cancer.

Name   What would make visiting
                                            enjoyable for him or her?

_____

_____

_____

_____

_____

_____

_____

_____

_____

_____

_____

_____

_____

_____

_____

_____

_____

_____

_____

_____

_____

_____

(Use extra sheets of paper, if necessary.)

"My wife loves to talk about personal things that happen to people. So does her friend Mary. When we get together with Mary, they both talk about the people they know. Mary has a great time and so does my wife."

"Joe's not a great talker, so I arrange for him to be doing something when we get together. Sometimes it's cutting up food for the meal; sometimes it's playing cards with Dad. But it gives him something to do when he's with Dad, and this makes him feel comfortable about not talking all the time."

"Nancy is into fancy cooking. She's a great cook and she really appreciates a meal that takes some effort. So, when Nancy visits, I fix something special to eat. It's a way of saying 'thanks for coming' that Nancy understands."

"Bill has a lot of problems of his own, so, when we visit him, my wife and I spend a lot of time listening to him talk about his problems. Sometimes we can help him, but mostly we help by listening. Bill likes an audience, and my wife and I don't mind listening—it makes us think our problems aren't really so bad."

"Judy is embarrassed if you thank her for coming. She likes to pretend that she was just passing by. So Andy and I play along. When I see her after church, I tell her how much her visits mean to Andy. Then I can tell she's pleased."

Possible Obstacles

Think about what could prevent you from carrying out your plan. Here are some things that other people have said stood in their way in carrying out their plans to increase companionship for the person with cancer.

1. "People should volunteer to visit without being asked."

   Response: If you feel this way, think back to people you knew who were sick and how difficult it sometimes was to find the time to visit. <u>The fact that people don't volunteer doesn't mean that they don't care</u>. Probably they would welcome the opportunity to visit—if they were asked.

2. "I'm afraid I'll be turned down if I invite people or if I ask to visit them."

   Response: Think of yourself as asking for the person who is sick and not for yourself. This way you are not so personally involved. <u>If you ask people to do something they enjoy doing, it is more likely that they will accept</u>.

3. "Some people feel awkward talking to someone who is sick. They don't know what to say."

   Response: <u>Have something to do—for example, a card game or puzzle to work on</u>. Then they can talk about what they are doing, or they can be comfortable not talking at all because they are paying attention to what they are doing.

4. "The person I am caring for says he doesn't want people to see him when he is sick."

   Response: Encourage talking to people on the phone. You may also suggest inviting people who are used to seeing sick people—for example, people who have been caring for someone who is sick. <u>You can also arrange activities that the visitors enjoy so that the appearance of the person with cancer isn't as important.</u>

5. "Some people are well meaning, but they boss us around or say things that are upsetting."

   Response: Well-meaning people are not always helpful, so think carefully about when their visits are helpful and when they are not. Invite them when their helpfulness outweighs any problems they cause. <u>If you and the person with cancer know what to expect and are prepared, you can steer the conversation in helpful directions during the visit.</u>

6. "Some people stay too long and tire us out."

   Response: <u>Ask them beforehand to limit the time they stay</u>. This takes the pressure off of everyone about when to end the visit.

Think of *other* obstacles that could interfere with carrying out your plan

What additional road blocks could get in the way of doing the things recommended in this home care plan? For example, will the person with cancer cooperate? Will other people help? How will you explain your needs to other people? Do you have the time and energy to carry out the plan?

You need to develop plans for getting around these road blocks. Use the four COPE ideas (creativity, optimism, planning, and expert information) in developing your plans. See the chapter on Solving Home Care Problems at the beginning of the book for a discussion of how to use the four COPE ideas in overcoming your obstacles.

Carrying out your plan

Make up a list of people who can give companionship. Keep adding ideas for how to make visiting pleasant and rewarding for them. Try new people. Don't just stick with the easy ones.

Invite people to come to visit the person with cancer or go to visit them. If you are uncomfortable inviting other people, ask others to do the inviting for you. Use the telephone to visit and encourage others to call. <u>Set deadlines to do this, or you may put it aside</u>.

Checking on results

You will know if your plans for companionship are successful by the number of times—either in person or on the phone—that the person with cancer is meeting other people.

If the plan does not work

Don't be discouraged if you are not completely successful in the beginning. You will become better with practice. <u>Start with people who are easier to visit or invite and gradually try people who are more challenging</u>.

If you are having problems, ask other people to help you and to give you ideas. When you are under pressure, it may be more difficult to reach out to others. If so, ask others to help you.

<u>You should repeat these problem-solving steps regularly throughout the illness to ensure that the person you are caring for has the companionship he or she wants and needs</u>.

Problems with Getting Information from Medical Staff

Overview of the Home Care Plan for
Problems with Getting Information from Medical Staff

Understanding the Problem

Getting medical information can be difficult

Each medical organization has different rules for who can give information

You have to learn the rules for each new treatment setting

What information to ask for

Getting Information in an Emergency

If you feel the situation is an emergency, call the doctor and use the word "emergency" in your request for information

Improving Your Ability To Get Information

Be sure your questions are phrased clearly

Learn who can answer your questions

Ask the person yourself or have someone ask for you

Possible Obstacles

"My questions are stupid."

"I feel confused by the health care system."

"I feel intimidated by medical staff."

"If I need to know something, the doctor will tell me."

"If I ask too many questions, the staff will think I'm a nuisance, and they won't take good care of the person I'm helping."

Carrying Out and Adjusting Your Plan

Ask questions—practice beforehand

Keep track of the problems you are having

If you feel you are not getting the information you need, talk to the physician about your problem

Get help from a "patient advocate" at the hospital

As a last resort, the person with cancer can change doctors

Kinds of Information that Different Medical Professions Can Usually Give You

(Topics with an arrow in front of them are actions you can take or symptoms you can look for.)

Problems with Getting Information from Medical Staff

Understanding the Problem

Over the course of the illness, you will need a great deal of information to do your job as family caregiver correctly. Some of this information is complicated, and often it must come from different sources. Therefore, it is not surprising that many family caregivers experience problems at some time during the illness with getting information that they need. This home care plan helps you deal with this problem by showing you an orderly sequence of steps to go through in getting medical information.

There are two things you should understand about getting medical information:

1. <u>It is usually reasonable to assume that the medical staff wants to help you and would like to give you the information you need.</u>

2. <u>Often certain staff members can't answer your questions because each medical care organization has its own rules about who knows what and who is allowed to give information to patients and caregivers.</u> One doctor's office has different rules from another doctor's office. One hospital differs from another, and, even within the same hospital, there are often different rules for inpatient (patients who stay overnight) and outpatient (patients who come and go in the same day) departments, different rules in surgery and in oncology, and so on. What this means is that you have to learn who knows what and who can tell you what for each new office, service, or hospital that you deal with.

What information should you ask for?

As a family caregiver, you should have all the information you need to provide the best possible care at home. The five kinds of information in the home care plans should always be available to you: an understanding of the problem (What is the problem? What causes it? Who is most likely to have the problem? What can family caregivers expect to accomplish in dealing with the problem?); when to call for professional help; what you can do to deal with and prevent the problem; obstacles that might interfere with your dealing with the problem; and how to carry out and monitor your plan. You need *all* of this information if you are to meet your caregiving responsibilities, and you should feel free to ask for information and to persist until you have it.

Your goal in using this home care plan is to get medical information that you need as quickly and efficiently as possible and with as little stress as possible for yourself and for medical staff with whom you deal.

Getting Information in an Emergency

Who to call for help

If you feel the situation is an emergency and you cannot get the information you need, then you should call the doctor or an emergency room. Be sure the person to whom you speak understands that you feel this is an emergency. To do this, use the word "emergency" in your question, and then be persistent until you have the information you need.

Here are some examples of phrasing you might use:

I have an emergency and need to talk to a doctor. (Be prepared to answer the question "What is the emergency?")

I have a question about _____ and I'm not sure if this is really an emergency or not. Who can help me?

I'm very concerned about _____. I think it may be an emergency. Can you help me?

Improving Your Ability To Get Information

There are three things you can do to improve your ability to get information you need. We recommend that you do the steps in this order:

1. Be sure your questions are phrased clearly.

2. Learn who can answer your questions.

3. Ask the person yourself or have someone ask for you.

Be sure that your questions are phrased clearly

Know exactly what information you need, and state your questions clearly.

➤ **Ask yourself "What do I need to know to do my job as a home caregiver?"** This question is one of the best ways to begin deciding what other questions to ask to give you information that you need. This focuses your attention on what is most important. Otherwise, you may find yourself asking a lot of questions without finding out what you really need to know.

➤ **When you ask questions, first say what you need to know and why you need to know it.** It is much easier for someone else to understand your question if you start with a clear statement of the information you need. Then your listener will be able to understand the rest of what you say. For example, let's assume that the person you are caring for had malaria when he was in the service. You noticed that some of the symptoms after chemotherapy were similar to malaria, and this made you worried that the malaria was returning. When you ask your question start by asking if any of his symptoms could be due to malaria. Say that the reason you are concerned is that he had malaria when he was in the service, and the symptoms after chemotherapy are very similar. The listener then knows both what you want to know and why. On the other hand, if you started with a long tale about his being in the South Pacific during the Second World War, and that he got malaria there, and that it almost killed him, and finally got around to asking what this has to do with his chemotherapy symptoms, the listener could be confused. He or she might think, "Is she telling me about his service record because she wants me to know what a hero he was? Or because she thinks malaria may have caused his cancer? Or because malaria and chemotherapy symptoms are similar?" As you can see, it is much clearer to the listener if you start with what you need to know.

➤ **Write out your questions and check them with other people.** Writing down your questions beforehand is one of the best ways to be sure you are being clear. Having a nurse or social worker read your list before you see your doctor is a good way to check on your clarity. If you get flustered, which happens to many people, then you can read your questions.

Learn who can answer your questions

Different people can give you different kinds of information, and this can vary with different doctors, hospitals, and clinics. You need to know who can tell you what for each new treatment setting.

➤ **Learn which staff members give different kinds of information to patients.** The best way to find this out is to ask a medical staff person such as a nurse, social worker, or physician. Secretarial staff are less likely to know this, but sometimes they can be of help. Nurses or social workers are usually aware of these rules. A good way to ask is to start your question with "who can tell me . . . " For example, "Who can tell me when my husband will be discharged" or "Who can tell me when my mother's treatments are scheduled?"

<u>Be prepared to learn the rules about who can give you what information for every new group of health staff that you deal with</u>. It is a good idea to ask these questions early, when you begin working with a new treatment team. That way you can avoid information problems later.

Be persistent! If medical staff say they don't know or can't tell you, then ask who can. You may have to ask several people, but don't feel that you are getting the run-around. Medical care is often complicated, which means that getting information about it can be complicated, too. Don't get discouraged. You have a right to all of the information you need to be the best possible caregiver. Pleasant persistence almost always pays off. Getting information becomes easier and easier the better you understand the medical care system.

(See the last page of this home care plan for a list of the types of information that different professional groups can usually give you.)

Ask the person yourself or have someone ask for you

➤ **Ask the question yourself.** Have a clear idea of what you need to know. Ask or read your questions. <u>Ask follow-up questions until you are very clear about the answer you received</u>.

➤ **Ask a nurse, social worker, or other member of the health care team to get the information you need.** You may need to ask someone else to get information for you because you don't have the time to find the right person. It could be because the medical person you need to talk to is not available when you need the information, or it could be that he or she gives you an answer, but the answer doesn't contain the information you need. If any of these things happen, a good strategy is to ask a nurse or social worker to ask your questions for you. <u>Nurses and social workers understand medical terminology and how medical organizations work. They are also usually good at explaining these things to nonmedical people</u>. Choose nurses or social workers with whom you feel comfortable, and tell them what information you need and why you can't get it yourself. Then ask for their help.

➤Ask the person with cancer to get the information you need.
The person with cancer sees all the people on the health care team and can be helpful in getting information that you need as a caregiver. However, people with cancer may have other things on their minds when they see the members of their health care team, so you may want to write down your questions, and you may also want to ask one of the staff (such as a nurse or social worker) to remind the person with cancer to ask the questions.

Sometimes the person with cancer doesn't want to ask questions because the answers may be upsetting. In this case, you should ask the questions yourself.

Possible Obstacles

What could prevent you from carrying out your plan to improve your ability to get information you need?

1. "My questions are stupid."

   Response: No questions are stupid. You and the medical staff want to give the best possible care to the person with cancer. For this to happen, you must understand what you need to do and why. Therefore, it is the medical staff's job to educate and inform you.

2. "I feel confused by the health care system."

   Response: Medical staff use unfamiliar words, have peculiar titles, and are organized into groups with unfamiliar names. It is not surprising that many patients and their families are confused. It can be almost as confusing as going to a foreign country. What many people do when they go to a foreign country is to get a guide who speaks their language and the language of the new country. This is a good model for learning about the health care system. Your guides can be health care staff who know the system—nurses and social workers are often good guides. Ask them to explain the system to you: what the titles mean, what the different groups do, and what medical terms mean. As you learn about the system, you will soon be using the medical terms yourself and finding your way around like a veteran.

3. "I feel intimidated by medical staff."

Response: Some people feel that medical staff are so important or so busy that they should not take up their valuable time with questions. This attitude is wrong. <u>Medical staff are there to help patients</u>. To do this, the staff must give family caregivers the information they need to care for the person with cancer at home.

4. "If I need to know something, the doctor will tell me."

Response: Not necessarily true! <u>Although your doctor will try to tell you everything you need to know, he or she can't always remember what you were told before, may assume that someone else told you, or may simply forget to tell you certain things</u>.

5. "If I ask too many questions, the staff will think I'm a nuisance, and then they won't take good care of the person I am helping."

Response: It is unlikely that the staff will think you are a nuisance, but, even if they do, <u>there is no reason to fear that this would affect how they treat the person with cancer</u>. Medical professionals are trained to treat everyone to the best of their ability no matter what they think about the person. To do otherwise would be malpractice.

Think of *other* obstacles that could interfere with carrying out your plan

What additional road blocks could get in the way of doing the things recommended in this home care plan? For example, how will you find time to get the information you need? How will you ask other people to help? What if they refuse? Will the person with cancer cooperate?

You need to develop plans for getting around your road blocks. Use the four COPE ideas (creativity, optimism, planning, and expert information) in developing your plans. See the chapter on Solving Home Care Problems at the beginning of the book for a discussion of how to use the four COPE ideas in overcoming your obstacles.

Carrying Out and Adjusting Your Plan

Carrying out your plan

Ask questions. <u>The more questions you ask, the easier it becomes</u>. In the beginning you may want to read your questions. Also practice beforehand what you will say. Set deadlines for getting certain information.

Checking on results

Keep track of the number of times you have problems getting information you need. Don't expect perfect results right away. However, over time you should notice significant improvement in your ability to get the information you need.

If your plan doesn't work

1. If you are having some success, but not as much as you would like, you may be expecting too much progress too soon. Be patient and keep trying. The medical care system is complicated, and it takes time to master it.

2. If you feel that medical staff are not giving you the information you need, your next step should be to make an appointment with the physician who has responsibility for the patient's care at that time and ask him or her your questions. You should also explain the problems you have had in getting information and ask how to avoid these problems in the future.

   (Note that you may be charged for this appointment, and many insurers will not pay for appointments with carepersons. It is best to ask about this when making the appointment. If you cannot afford to pay, you can ask to have the fee waived or you can ask if your meeting can be scheduled as part of the patient's regular meeting with the physician.)

   Don't be angry and don't be intimidated. Being angry only makes the other person angry, too, and being intimidated means that you won't explain the situation clearly. A calm, objective approach works best.

3. Most hospitals have patient advocates or similar staff members. These people are familiar with problems in the hospital as well as with how to deal with those problems. They can help you to get information, and, in addition, they can help to change the way the hospital operates. You may help future patients by telling patient advocates about problems you are having.

4. As a last resort, the person with cancer always has the right to change doctors or treatment settings. If he or she is considering that, be sure that the new setting will give the support you need.

Kinds of Information that Different Medical Professions Can Usually Give You

<u>Physicians</u>: treatment plans, prognosis (the likelihood of cure or remission and the usual course of the disease), how often the patient will be evaluated, how often he or she needs to see a doctor, when he or she should be admitted to a hospital, what medicines should be taken and when, results of tests, and whether the medicine is working.

<u>Nurses</u>: management of side effects of treatments, appointment schedules, nutrition information, results of some tests (this depends on the doctor or hospital policies), how and when to take medications not prescribed by a doctor.

<u>Social workers</u>: help in dealing with family and emotional problems, how to arrange for medical care at home, how to be admitted to a nursing home or hospice program, how to get financial help or whether you qualify for different government programs.

This list is a good starting point for getting information, but be prepared for lots of exceptions. Hospital physicians have different titles such as "attending," "fellow," "resident," and "consultant" as well as different types of specialties such as "surgeon," "oncologist," "radiotherapist," "pathologist," and so on. Depending on your medical needs, physicians with different titles and specialties have different responsibilities and can give you different kinds of information. When several physicians are involved, one member of the team will be coordinating the care. In this case, ask who the coordinating physician is.

Getting Help from Community Agencies and Volunteer Groups

Overview of the Home Care Plan for
Getting Help from Community Agencies and Volunteer Groups

Understanding the Problem

Many people struggle alone with their problems when there are people and agencies in their communities able and willing to help

Knowing about these services is like having "money in the bank" that you can use when you need it

Learn about these services *before* you need them

When To Get Professional Help

If you are having difficulty arranging for the help you need, ask to speak to a social worker

What You Can Do To Get Help

Getting help in finding community services

Transportation and driving

Home nursing services

Hospice care

Help with meals and household chores

Paying hospital or medical expenses

Possible Obstacles

"If people want to help, they'll offer."

"I'm afraid I'll be turned down."

"No one is available to help with driving."

"I hold back on help to save my insurance benefits."

"I feel embarrassed not being able to pay my bills."

"I didn't handle the money in our family."

Carrying Out and Adjusting Your Plan

Don't wait—start learning now before you need help

It takes time to learn to use community resources

If you are feeling too worn down to get help, ask someone such as a social worker to help you—this is his or her specialty

(Topics with an arrow in front of them are actions you can take or symptoms you can look for.)

Getting Help from Community Agencies and Volunteer Groups

Understanding the Problem

Many people with cancer and their families do not fully understand the services that are available to help them in their own communities and in the hospitals and clinics where they receive treatment. As a result, they struggle alone with their problems when there are people and organizations able and willing to help. Finding out about these services and how to qualify for and use them is a challenge.

Even if you don't need to use these services right now, knowing that they are available is like having "money in the bank." It can reassure you that there are resources available to help when you need them.

This home care plan discusses five types of services that persons with cancer sometimes need and that are available in most communities: help with transportation and driving, home nursing visits, help with meals and household chores, hospice care for advanced cancer, and help paying for medical or hospital expenses. Understanding how to find and use these services will give you skills that you can use to find additional community services.

We recommend that you learn about available services *before* problems arise. You can do a more complete job of learning about these services when you are not under pressure to deal with a serious problem. If you need these services later, you will know what to do and where to go immediately.

Your goals are to:

know who to ask about community services,

what services are available in your community or hospital, and

how to qualify for and use those services.

When To Get Professional Help

If you are having difficulty arranging for the help you need, ask to speak to a social worker. Social workers are the professionals who are experienced in finding help from community agencies and volunteer groups.

Most hospitals have social workers on their staff, so you can ask a doctor or nurse at the hospital where the person with cancer is receiving treatment to arrange for you to talk to a social worker.

What You Can Do To Get Help

Getting help in finding community services

There are four places you can go for help in finding and using services in the community. We suggest that you try all of these since one may list something that others do not. They are:

➤ **Hospital social workers.** They are professionals with knowledge, skills, and experience in finding community services to help patients and their families deal with illness-related problems. They deal regularly with community agencies and know not only what services are available, but also which agencies provide the best services. You are entitled to talk to social workers when the person with cancer is a patient in the hospital or is coming for treatments at the hospital. Usually you can call the social workers directly without being referred, but in some hospitals they prefer that the doctor make a referral. To get a referral, tell the doctor or nurse that you want to talk to a social worker.

➤ **"Knowledgeable people" in your community.** People in certain positions in a community know a lot about which local agencies and organizations provide services. Clergy are usually well informed on these matters as well as local elected officials and officers of local community organizations such as the United Way. If these people can't help you directly, they usually know who to ask.

➤ **Agencies that help you find services.** Most communities have agencies that specialize in helping people find the services they need. They have different titles in different communities or parts of the country, but some examples are local offices of the American Cancer Society, United Way, Area Agencies for the Aging, religious agencies such as Catholic Charities or the local Councils of Churches, and community mental health centers. Hospital social workers know about these agencies in your area and can explain what they do.

➤ **The "Guide to Human Services" section of local telephone books.** Most local telephone books contain sections listing community agencies and the services they provide. Often this is in a separate section and is printed on a different color paper to set it off from the rest. Often the pages are blue. Look at the table of contents in the beginning of your local telephone book for the Guide to Human Services or a similar title.

Transportation and driving

Getting transportation to and from treatments or medical appointments can be difficult. You should look for help if any of the following conditions exist:

1. You cannot drive the person to appointments.
2. You cannot get the person from the house to the car or they cannot sit for the length of the trip.
3. You are falling asleep at the wheel, the trip is too long, you hesitate to drive, or you fear the trip.
4. You cannot miss work or give up the money from work hours to take the time needed for the trip, the waiting, the appointment, and the return trip.

<u>There are several things you can do to solve these transportation problems.</u>

➤ **Ask family or friends for help with driving.** <u>The more specific you are, the more likely that others will understand your request and be able to judge what is involved with their service.</u> Tell them:

> What days of the week you could use drivers
>
> How long the trip takes each way
>
> Whether he or she can be dropped off
>
> Whether someone will meet him or her at the door
>
> How much parking costs
>
> How long the usual appointment lasts
>
> Whether he or she needs help getting in and out
>
> Whether a wheelchair is involved
>
> Whether money is available for their gasoline expenses

➤ **Ask a family member or a friend to arrange transportation.** If you don't want to ask for help, have someone else ask for you. If someone else sets up the schedule, then you are freer from worry and telephone calls about dates and times. Having a scheduler is especially helpful when the person with cancer must go for treatments every day or every week. Church groups often arrange transportation for members and may be willing to arrange drivers for nonmembers.

➤ **Ask the American Cancer Society if they have a volunteer transportation program.** Many offices of the American Cancer Society run transportation programs through their Service and Rehabilitation Committee. Volunteer drivers are trained to help the person with cancer, and their service is free. In addition, the schedule of drivers is arranged for you. If your local office does not have such a program, then ask if the next nearest office has a transportation program. Sometimes volunteer drivers who live close to your county are willing to help with driving.

➤ **Call the American Cancer Society to find out if you are eligible to receive partial reimbursement for gas.** The Cancer Society can give you partial reimbursement for gas and expenses, if you are eligible. Save receipts to give to them. There is a monthly or yearly limit to the amount of money reimbursed, but the Cancer Society sometimes extends this limit in situations of extreme need.

➤ **Ask local service clubs, such as the Elks, Lions Club, Masons, or American Legion if they or their auxiliaries could schedule drivers or help with transportation expenses.** There are several organizations that have volunteers who drive people with serious illnesses to medical appointments. This varies from community to community. Check with your local organizations. Ask the club or their auxiliaries to assign one member to schedule drivers. Some service groups raise money to help with medical expenses. If a relative or friend belongs to such a group in your community, ask them to explain your needs.

➤ **Ask a social worker, caseworker, or nurse to recommend paid drivers to you.** Do not try to get paid help on your own. Ask the social worker or nurse involved in caring for the patient for guidance in finding paid help. They understand the kind of help you need, and they have had experience with different agencies and ways to get help.

➤ **Ask if the treatment center or medical clinic has their own transportation van service.** Some centers offer free transportation to and from chemotherapy or radiation appointments. Usually these are van services, and the person must be prepared to spend half the day at the treatment site. Many enjoy riding with others who are receiving similar treatments.

➤ **Use the county medical van.** If treatments are within the county, the county van service may help you. If treatments are outside of the county, ask if the transportation service crosses county lines.

Home nursing services

There are three types of nursing services: visits from registered nurses, visits from private duty nurses, and visits from nurses' aides.

➤ **Visits from registered nurses.** The doctor can prescribe home visits by registered nurses to do skilled nursing procedures and to give certain chemotherapy drugs at home. They can come to the home for short procedures, such as taking blood or urine samples to the laboratory for you or helping with dressing changes on a wound, ostomy opening, or intravenous (IV) site. Nurses can come out once a week or every day to do "skilled nursing procedures," such as teaching how to care for an IV line, how to change a dressing on a wound, or how to take medicines correctly. Their visits are often short (about an hour), and the cost is covered by insurance after they get approval from a doctor to visit. They also can arrange for others to visit, if needed, such as nurses' aides, social workers, speech therapists, occupational therapists, and physical therapists.

Some agencies send a nurse out just to do a blood draw or some other short task. The cost of this visit is seldom covered by insurance, but the fees are low. Ask the nurses or social workers to recommend an agency you can call to talk about this option.

Chemotherapy nurses can come to the home when it is difficult to travel to the clinic. These nurses can be the same ones you see at the clinic or doctor's office where chemotherapy is given, or they can be employed by a visiting nurse agency. Ask the clinic nurses about this possibility.

➤ **Visits from private-duty nurses.** You can arrange for private-duty nurses without a doctor's approval. Visits from these nurses can last as long as you want. For example, some families find it helpful to arrange for 8 hours of overnight care. The cost of this service is usually not covered by insurance, but be sure to ask in case it is.

➤ **Visits from nurses' aides.** You can arrange for nurses' aides for personal care services without a doctor's approval. Nurses' aides can visit when you do not need help from a registered nurse. Sometimes agencies have a sliding scale fee because the state or county has given them money to provide "personal care services" in the home. Nurses' aides, also called attendants, can help with bathing, walking, shopping, cooking, and light household chores.

Hospice care

Hospice care is used for advanced cancer, when quality of life rather than lengthening life is the goal of care. Ask the social worker or nurse about hospice care in your community.

Hospice teams help people with life-limiting or terminal illnesses. Their services are available in all cities and most small towns and rural areas. Hospices are often run by the local visiting nurse agencies, and their visits are covered by insurance. Nurses and social workers at the hospital or clinics know who to call about hospice care, and a hospice worker can come talk with you about their many services, including helping you manage pain.

Help with meals and household chores

➤**Look up "Meals" in the phone book and ask about home-delivered meals,** or call your local Area Agency on the Aging, which will be listed in the phone book. Most cities and small towns have home-delivered meals. Many of these programs are for senior citizens. If you are under 65 years old, you may still be able to qualify, so call and ask. The cost of the service varies, and you may be eligible for reduced rates. Usually a hot lunch is delivered with a cold meal to be eaten later in the day. Special diets are available, such as diabetic, low-sodium, and low-fat diets. If these services are not listed under "Meals" in the phone book, look for the Area Agency on the Aging, which often provides these services or knows who does.

➤**Ask about agencies that help with meal preparation.** Some agencies have programs where a worker or nurses' aide comes to the home a few times a week for 1 to 2 hours. They can shop for food and supplies, run errands, prepare meals, and do light housekeeping.

➤**Ask church groups or neighbors to organize a small home helper group.** Many churches are happy to do this and can do yard work, window washing, or other chores. Sometimes they arrange for the youth group to get involved.

Paying medical or hospital expenses

It is important that you deal with financial problems early—before they become a crisis. Don't put it off. The earlier you start working on this problem, the easier it will be to solve. If you talk to the people you owe money to before it becomes a crisis, they are usually willing to work with you. Following is a list of things that you can do to help solve this problem.

➤**Collect the facts.** The first thing you should do is to collect information about the expenses you have now and expect to have in the future as well as about your financial resources. You need this information to decide what help you need and qualify for, and, if you do ask for help, you will be asked for this information.

➤ Figure out your medical expenses.

1. How much do you now owe for medical expenses? This is often difficult to know, especially with the confusing way that many hospitals and other health care organizations send their bills. Most hospitals and doctors' offices have someone on their staff who understands the billing forms. These people can quickly go through a stack of bills and determine exactly what you owe at that time.

2. What future expenses do you anticipate?

3. Approximately how much have you paid out so far for medical care during this illness? Keep track of your medical expenses that are not covered by insurance since they may be deductible from your income taxes. This information will help you show others that you need financial assistance.

➤ Figure out what your financial resources are.

1. What kind of medical expenses does your insurance pay and not pay? This is important information to have even before your bills arrive. It helps you to estimate what your expenses will be. Ask your insurance agent or your health insurance representative where you or the person with cancer works.

2. What are your savings?

3. What do you own (house, property, stocks)?

4. What is the total income of your household? Household income is the total income of everyone living in the same household with the person with cancer. This information is often used to calculate if you are eligible for financial assistance.

➤ Investigate spacing out paying bills or paying in installments. To help with this, contact the financial counselor or the business or credit office in the hospital. They can help you to set up a monthly payment plan. Some hospitals, doctors, and pharmacies submit bills to the insurance company and then bill you for what the insurance won't pay. This saves you from paying the bills and then waiting for reimbursement from the insurance company. Ask your hospital or doctor's office if they will do this.

➤ Investigate borrowing money. Banks and other organizations that lend money will want to know about your financial situation and about money you expect to receive in the future. Collect this information before you talk to them. Shop around for the best terms and the most reasonable interest.

➤ **Apply for financial help.** <u>Social workers are usually the best source of information about how to get help with medical expenses and who qualifies for help</u>. Most hospitals employ social workers, and, if the person you are caring for is a patient there, you can make an appointment with a social worker. However, if the hospital is far from your home, the hospital social worker may not be familiar with resources in your community. Following is a list of community services that you can explore.

Help with medication costs is sometimes available from the American Cancer Society (ACS). Call your local ACS office. Some drug companies also offer free medication programs. Ask the doctor or nurse if there are any drug company programs to help with your medication costs.

The Leukemia Society of America also sometimes helps with medication costs for adults and children with leukemia, lymphoma, or Hodgkin's disease.

People on disability, veterans, and people receiving vocational rehabilitation services often qualify for financial assistance for cancer treatments. Ask the social worker to check that you are receiving your benefits.

Other sources of financial help include the American Red Cross, county boards of assistance, and United Way agencies. Sometimes they will help with past expenses as well as future expenses. These agencies are listed in the white and blue pages of your telephone book. Hospital social workers will often help you find and apply for help from community organizations. You can either call the social work department yourself or ask the doctor or nurse to refer you to them.

Family, friends, and community groups can often help people in financial need because of illness. Some community groups have funds to help group members, but others, especially religious groups, have funds to help anyone in need. Talk to members of community organizations and churches about your needs.

Possible Obstacles

**Here are some things that others have said
stood in their way of using community services
or getting help with expenses**

1. "I don't want to ask for help. If people want to help, they'll offer."

   Response: Some people feel that their friends and relatives should volunteer to help without being asked. If you feel this way, think back to people you knew who were sick and how difficult it sometimes was to find the time or inclination to volunteer to help. <u>The fact that people don't volunteer doesn't mean that they would not help. Family and friends will probably welcome the opportunity to help if asked because they know that they are meeting a specific need</u>. The home care plan for Getting Companionship and Support from Family and Friends has ideas to make helping enjoyable for everyone.

2. "I'm afraid I'll be turned down."

   Response: Many people are not sure how to ask for help, and they may be afraid that they will be turned down. If you feel this way, here is a suggestion. <u>Think of yourself as asking for the person who is sick and not for yourself</u>. You could also ask someone else to do the asking for you.

3. "No one around here can help drive. They don't have the time or the money for gas. Some don't even have cars or they work or are too busy with their families."

   Response: <u>You don't know who can drive until you ask</u>. Ask other people to help you find drivers. Also, retirees and those who are temporarily unemployed might have the time to give to help you solve this problem.

4. "I hold back on getting treatments or services because I don't want to use up my insurance benefits."

   Response: <u>Now is the time to use your benefits—when you have a serious illness</u>. There are some policies with maximum benefits, but these are usually very large and will more than cover the costs of cancer treatments. Check your insurance policy to be sure.

5. "I feel embarrassed and humiliated not to be able to pay my bills."

   Response: Many people, just like yourself, have been in the same situation. Medical expenses are so large today that it is becoming common for many people to have problems paying them. <u>You should not feel embarrassed since the problem is not your fault</u>. You will find that almost everyone is very understanding.

6. "I didn't handle money in our family—other people did—so I don't know what to do."

   Response: <u>If money matters are new to you, then get help from someone who is familiar with budgets and paying bills</u>. Don't let things drift because they can get out of hand and you will have a financial crisis to deal with.

**Think of *other* obstacles that could interfere
with carrying out your plan**

What additional road blocks could get in the way of doing the things recommended in this home care plan? For example, can you get the financial information you need? Do you know where your financial records are kept? Can you understand financial records? How will you explain your needs to other people? Do you have the time and energy to carry out the plan?

You need to develop plans for getting around your road blocks. Use the four COPE ideas (creativity, optimism, planning, and expert information) in developing your plans. See the chapter on Solving Home Care Problems at the beginning of the book for a discussion of how to use the four COPE ideas in overcoming your obstacles.

Carrying Out and Adjusting Your Plan

How will you carry out your plan?

Don't wait! Start learning *now* before you need information about how community agencies and volunteer groups can help you. This will be valuable information that you can use when you need it. If you have trouble getting the information you need, ask someone to help you. Talk to a social worker at the hospital. They have had a great deal of experience with these problems and can often be creative in helping you to get the help you need.

If your plan doesn't work

If you are having some success but not as much as you would like, you may be expecting too much progress too soon. Be patient and keep trying. It often takes time to learn how to use community agencies and volunteer groups.

If you are feeling worn down by your problems, ask someone else to help you work out a solution. Sometimes people who are not directly involved can see new ways to deal with the problem.

Social workers are the professionals who have the most experience with these problems. If the social worker to whom you talked was not helpful, ask to talk to another social worker.

Moving around the House

Overview of the
Home Care Plan for Moving around the House

Understanding the Problem

Mobility problems are a challenge

You have to learn what equipment is available to help and how to use it to best advantage

When To Get Professional Help

Situations and symptoms requiring professional help and how to get it

What to say when you call

What You Can Do To Help

Increase safety during walking or moving

Check to see if you can receive reimbursement

Locate medical equipment for use in the home

Possible Obstacles

"The person I'm caring for won't use the things I arrange to help him get around."

Carrying Out and Adjusting Your Plan

Develop your plan with the person you are caring for

Only buy equipment if it can't be borrowed or rented

Keep track of problems

If problems continue, ask a social worker or nurse for help

(Topics with an arrow in front of them are actions you can take or symptoms you can look for.)

Moving around the House

[The information in this home care plan fits most situations, but yours may be different.

If the doctor or nurse tells you to do something else, follow what they say. If you think there may be a medical emergency, see pages 211–212.]

Understanding the Problem

People with cancer can experience a variety of physical problems at different times during the course of treatment and over the length of illness. One problem that is particularly discouraging and potentially unsafe is when they have difficulty moving about, keeping balanced, bathing, or getting up from different pieces of furniture because of feeling slowed down or weak.

Helping with transfers in the bathroom or around the home can be an added challenge to many caregivers. Some caregivers have bad backs or health problems of their own that prohibit lifting or straining. Others who are sometimes away from the home have the additional worry that the person with cancer in a weaker state could fall. Caregivers can become frustrated when assisting a taller or heavier person.

<u>Many pieces of equipment and safety tips can make moving around, bathing, and transfers safer and easier for both of you. It's a matter of learning what is available and how to use the necessary equipment to the best advantage.</u>

Your goals are to:

call for help if there is an emergency,

locate and use equipment that helps with moving around in the home,

receive reimbursement, where possible, for expenses, and

increase safety during walking or moving.

When To Get Professional Help

<u>You should call the social worker or nurse where the person with cancer is receiving treatment if any of the following conditions exist</u>:

➤**You are not able to help the person get from one piece of furniture to another.**

➤**You are not able to get the person from the house to the car.**

Moving Around

> The person has fallen repeatedly or been hurt in falling.

> The person with cancer needs oxygen all the time, and it is difficult for you to help him or her move around with the oxygen equipment.

Here is an example of what to tell a social worker or nurse about this problem when any of these things are true

"I am Mary Smith, the wife of Harold Smith. He fell today and he's having trouble getting off of his favorite couch. I'm afraid that he is going to hurt himself."

What You Can Do To Help

There are three things you can do on your own to help the person with cancer to move safely and comfortably:

increase safety during walking or moving,

receive reimbursement for expenses, and

locate medical equipment for use in the home.

Increase safety during walking and moving

> **Inspect the bathroom and stairs for safety.** Most accidents happen in these two places.

> **Install handrails in the shower or tub.** Many people hang onto towel racks for steadiness. However, towel racks can weaken and be pulled down. Handrails can be placed over the sides of tubs or installed directly into walls or shower stalls. Different sizes and widths are available in any home care catalog.

> **Place nonslip appliqués on the tub floor.** These can be purchased at most pharmacies, supermarkets, or hardware stores and decrease chances of slipping while showering or getting in and out of a tub.

> **Remove loose rugs.** Rugs are easy to slip on and should be removed, especially from linoleum and wooden floor surfaces.

> **Use a steady shower chair in the bathtub.** Shower chairs make bathing or showering much safer. The larger the chair, the steadier it is. Some shower chairs even stretch over the side of the tub so a person can sit on the bench and slide over to the tub without too much lifting or shifting of body weight. Many types of chairs are shown in home care catalogs.

➤ **Use wheelchairs or commodes with lift-off arms.** When these chairs have a lift-off arm, they can be positioned alongside a bed or couch, and a person can lift the arm off and easily slide over to the new seat.

➤ **Raise beds, toilets, chairs, and couches to make it easier to move on and off of them.** If the height of a bed is low, getting out of it can be difficult. The bed can be raised on wooden blocks for a safer and easier transfer. Toilets are often too low, and a raised toilet seat can be purchased to elevate it anywhere from 4 to 6 inches. Chairs and couches can be dangerously low and lead to strains and even fractures when one is trying to rise out of them. Again, wooden blocks can be placed under furniture to raise it to safer heights.

➤ **Try sliding boards between seats to help with awkward transfers.** Sliding boards are short pieces of wood that stretch between a wheelchair, for example, and a bed. The person does not have to stand to get from one place to another but shimmies across the board to the new setting. These are particularly helpful for tall people, for days when the person is feeling weak, for times when no one is there to help him or her move, and for caregivers with bad backs who can't lift or help the person switch places.

➤ **Consider using Lifeline™, a telephone service, to get help from neighbors.** Lifeline™ is a button that is worn around the neck or placed near the person with cancer, with which he or she can signal a neighbor for help. Most local community hospitals have this service for you to use. Look in the telephone book or call the hospital and ask for the Lifeline telephone number and contact person. Someone will interview you over the telephone and explain the monthly rental service. Sometimes financial discounts are available. You will need to name three neighbors who would agree to keep a key to the home and respond to a call from a central operator should the button be pushed. This system is an alternative to calling 911 or the emergency response unit.

Check to see if you can receive reimbursement or help with these expenses

➤ **Check if your insurance covers these expenses** *(many do not).*

➤ **Call the American Cancer Society to find out about your eligibility to receive partial reimbursement for equipment.** If you are financially eligible, the Cancer Society will help with some expenses, such as the rental of a Hoyer™ lift, which is a small hydraulic lift that moves a person from a bed to a chair or from a chair to another chair. The Cancer Society may also pay for other equipment or loan it to you.

➤ **Call organizations or groups that have raised money for medical expenses in the past and ask for help with expenses.** If you need an unusual piece of equipment and your insurance does not cover the rental or purchase, ask a service group for a donation. They are more likely to pay for equipment because they can see what their donation is being used for.

Locate medical equipment

➤ **Ask if the hospital or home care agency has their own supply stores.** Some have their own supply houses as well as personnel who will help you look at different options for home care.

➤ **Call a local medical equipment store to find out what they have to solve problems with moving.** Most medical supply stores can advise you on the telephone about options in equipment for use at home. Some are covered by insurance, and merchants usually know which pieces are covered with a doctor's prescription.

➤ **Pick up a home care catalog.** Many pharmacies and some large department stores with catalog services have catalogs that picture and describe a variety of home care equipment and devices.

➤ **Ask the American Cancer Society about donated equipment.** Some offices collect donated supplies that they will give to you to use at home.

➤ **Ask service groups about donated equipment.** Different service groups collect and repair equipment, such as wheelchairs and commodes. If a relative or friend belongs to a group that does this in your community, then ask them to approach the appropriate leaders, explain the need, and look over donated supplies.

Possible Obstacles

Here is an obstacle that others have said got in their way of solving problems with moving the person with cancer safely and comfortably

1. "The person I'm caring for won't use the things I arrange to help him get around."

   Response: If this is because he is confused, then you have to arrange for someone to be with him to be sure he does use the equipment. If this is because he does not want to acknowledge that he needs the equipment, then you need to involve him in developing and carrying out the plan. Remember that you should always involve the person you are caring for in your home care plans.

After all, it is his body and his feelings, so he has a right to be part of developing the plan. Being involved in the plan means that he agrees to what will be done. <u>You should discuss together what the problem is and what you will do to deal with it. If he does not agree that there is a problem for him, then explain how it is a problem for you.</u> Ask him to use the equipment for your sake. If he cannot understand your point of view, then get help from other people such as other family members, friends, or health professionals to help explain the problem to him.

If he does not want to have other people see him using the equipment, then put it away when there are guests. If he forgets to use the equipment, work out ways to remind him—for example, putting up signs—or you can practice using the equipment so that it becomes a habit.

Think of *other* obstacles that could interfere with carrying out your plan

What additional road blocks could get in the way of doing the things recommended in this home care plan? For example, will the person with cancer cooperate? Will other people help? How will you explain your needs to other people? Do you have the time and energy to carry out the plan?

You need to develop plans for getting around your road blocks. Use the four COPE ideas (creativity, optimism, planning, and expert information) in developing your plans. See the chapter on Solving Home Care Problems at the beginning of the book for a discussion of how to use the four COPE ideas in overcoming your obstacles.

Carrying Out and Adjusting Your Plan

Carrying out your plan

Develop your plan *with* the person you are caring for. <u>Try simpler solutions first—things you can do yourselves with what you have in your home.</u> Talk with nurses, social workers, physical therapists, or occupational therapists about your problems and ask for their suggestions. Look into borrowing equipment. If it can't be borrowed, look into renting if the equipment is going to be needed for a short time. Purchasing equipment can save money if it is needed for a long time.

Moving Around

Checking on results

Keep track of the problems he or she has in walking and moving. If a problem happens occasionally and it is not dangerous, you may want to wait to see if it becomes more frequent. If a problem is potentially dangerous and you are worried, then develop your plan before the problem becomes serious.

If your plan doesn't work

If your plan does not seem to be working or the problems in walking and moving are getting worse, there are two things you can do. Consider them in this order.

1. Check When To Get Professional Help in this care plan. If any of the conditions listed there exist, call the social worker or nurse immediately.

2. <u>If problems with moving around the house continue, ask the social worker or nurse for help</u>. Tell them what you have done and what the results have been.

Coordinating Care from One Treatment Setting to Another

Overview for the Home Care Plan for Coordinating Care from One Treatment Setting to Another

Understanding the Problem

People with cancer often spend time in several different treatment or care settings

When going from one setting to another, it is important to continue medication and care routines that have been successful

You should tell medical staff what works at home so that they can continue these routines in the new treatment setting

When To Get Professional Help

If it is an emergency or if you are not successful in coordinating care, then speak directly to the physician, head nurse, or patient advocate at the hospital where the person with cancer is receiving treatment

What You Can Do To Help

List the kinds of help that he or she needs

Ensure that his or her needs for medications, elimination, and maintaining familiar routines are met in the new setting

Possible Obstacles

"I expect the doctor to coordinate care."

"I don't want the staff to think I'm bossing them around."

Carrying Out and Adjusting Your Plan

Make lists before the transfer occurs

Check on whether plans are being followed

Involve the staff in solving problems with coordinating care

(Topics with an arrow in front of them are actions you can take or symptoms you can look for.)

Coordinating Care from One Treatment Setting to Another

Understanding the Problem

People with cancer are usually hospitalized more than once during different episodes of the illness, and they also may spend time in a rehabilitation center or nursing home. As you work out routines and schedules and learn to manage different symptoms and problems at home, you want to see many of these same routines followed as closely as possible whenever the person stays somewhere else.

Telling the health care staff what works at home helps them to deliver the best care no matter what the setting. Requesting that certain routines be followed increases the chances of continuing your home care plans successfully. If you don't inform the health care staff, particularly the admitting physician, about these needs, then the person with cancer may end up with unmanaged symptoms.

For example, if you and the person with cancer have settled on a schedule of pain pills that keeps the pain away and also keeps him or her fully alert, you don't want to see this regimen abandoned when he or she is hospitalized. This can happen, especially if the person is put in a different hospital from the one where the doctor who originally prescribed the pain medicine works. Another example of when schedules may be disrupted and symptoms mismanaged is when a different doctor prescribes additional doses of a pain medicine. The person with cancer might have been seen by medical oncologists for months but was seen later by a radiation oncologist and received a higher dose of pain medicine. If he or she returns to the medical oncologist, the new pain prescriptions need to be explained. Whoever admits the person to the hospital or any new setting needs to know exactly what drugs are given at home, when they are given, and how effective they are.

Maintaining medication schedules is not the only concern. Equipment that works well at home (such as a certain walker or toilet seat) should be used in the hospital or other setting. Personal care preferences and routines should also be known and followed, if possible.

Your goal is to:

continue helpful procedures and routines as the person with cancer moves from one treatment setting to another.

When To Get Professional Help

If the problems in coordinating care are making the person with cancer very uncomfortable, and you have tried the ideas in this plan without success, then ask to speak to a nurse supervisor or physician. Explain the problems you are having and why you are concerned, and ask for their help. If you still have problems, ask to talk to the patient advocate at the hospital. Patient advocates are on the staff of most hospitals, and their job is to help when you feel that the hospital is not doing its job.

What You Can Do To Help

The first thing you should do is to review the kinds of medical help, special equipment, diet, and other needs of the person with cancer. Then you should plan how you will ensure that these needs are met in the new treatment setting.

What kinds of help does the person with cancer need?

1. What kinds of medical help does he or she need?
   Help in taking medicines
   Help with medical procedures (such as ostomy or catheter care)
   Help with eating
   Help getting out of bed
   Help with walking
   Help going to the toilet
   Help with sleeping
   Help with bathing

2. Is any special equipment needed, such as a commode or foam eggshell mattress?

3. Is there a special diet to be followed?

4. What kinds of things make the day more enjoyable for him or her, such as listening to music, watching television, reading the newspaper, or getting the mail?

5. What does he or she worry about, and how can the staff be most comforting and reassuring?

6. What other facts would you want to tell to those who will be helping the person with cancer?

Plan how the needs of the person with cancer will be met in the new treatment setting

The person's needs can be grouped into two categories: continuing medical care and continuing familiar routines.

Continuing medical care in new treatment settings

Plan how you can continue the same schedule of medicines to prevent distressing symptoms or other discomforts.

➤ **Give a list to the admitting doctor or nurse of the names of and times of day that medicines are given.** This ensures that medicines are given close to the same times as usual. It is especially important to do this for medicines that were originally ordered as "prn" or "as needed," but you have learned that a certain timing or routine is most helpful—such as for pain medicines. If you tell this routine to the admitting physician and nurse, they can write orders so that the routine is changed as little as possible.

➤ **List the food or liquid that is served with the pills alongside the medicine schedule.** The staff can then copy the drug down on their charts as "give with milk" or "serve with small amount of applesauce." This makes it easier for the person with cancer to continue to take the medicines.

➤ **Write down in what form the pill is given**—for example, if it is crushed or mixed into applesauce. If pills are crushed, then they are crushed into something, such as Maalox™ or applesauce. Or a suppository may be used. If you write these instructions down, then there will be no confusion.

➤ **Ask that the admitting physician order a laxative or enema for the same day you would give one at home, if no bowel movement has occurred.** Unfortunately, it often takes a few days to notice constipation at a new setting. If the same elimination routine is followed there that is followed at home, less discomfort will result from this common problem.

➤ **Give a weekly schedule of elimination routines to the nurse.** At different times during an illness like cancer, complicated schedules need to be followed to prevent constipation or diarrhea. For example, if a soap suds enema on the third day without a bowel movement works well at home, then tell this to the nurse. This will make things easier for both the person you are caring for and for the nursing staff as well.

➤ **Ask the nurses to write the elimination plan in the nursing care plan.** Many times the family gives key information to the nurse who admits the person with cancer to the hospital or new setting, but it is written down in a long admission note, which may not be read by the nursing staff when problems occur. However, if this information is written on the nursing care plan or Kardex™, it will be noticed and used in caring for the patient.

➤ **Ask the nurses to order a bedside commode or raised toilet seat, if either is used at home.** Upon admission, the staff does not know how difficult it is for the person with cancer to get to the commode. If you used a bedside commode or a raised toilet seat at home, then it is likely they will be needed in the hospital, too. Tell the admitting physician or nurse about this so that the right equipment can be available when it is needed.

➤ **Ask the doctor to order a soft or blenderized diet, if it is preferred.** If the person with cancer needs or prefers a soft diet, then tell this to the admitting physician or nurse. This ensures that meals are edible, especially if a sore mouth or mouth ulcers are a problem.

➤ **Ask the doctor to write the mouth care regimen used at home in the admitting orders.** If warm salt rinses or baking soda rinses are a routine at home, then they should be part of the doctor's admitting orders. The staff will then give these items to the person and help with rinsing. Otherwise, it is up to you or the person with cancer to bring the salt or baking soda in and remember to rinse after meals and at bedtime.

Continuing familiar routines in new treatment settings

➤ **Bring the mail and newspaper.** Familiar routines are not limited to medicines and personal care. Staying in touch with one's home can also bring a sense of comfort and control.

➤ **Bring musical tapes, relaxation tapes, or radios that are used at home.** Distractions, no matter how short, are important for relief of anxiety or tension that goes along with being in the hospital or nursing center. Music or relaxation tapes can be brought in and played for enjoyment and distraction. Radios are not usually available in these settings, so you may have to bring one in for the person to listen to favorite news and music programs. Earphones should be used if he or she is in a semi-private room.

➤ **Bring turbans, scarves, caps, or head coverings worn at home.** Looking presentable can be very important to someone who is sick. Any head coverings used at home should also be an option here.

➤ **Bring in aids to walking, such as canes or walkers.**

➤ **Bring in aids to comfort and sleep, such as small pillows or favorite blankets.**

➤ **If a special mattress is needed, ask for it ahead of time.** Many people like the contour of eggshell mattresses. Other mattresses are ones filled with air or water, if skin care is a problem, or ones that alternate air pressure and gently inflate and deflate at different spots along the mattress. If a special mattress is used at home, ask that the same be used in the new setting. If you ask ahead of time, it's more likely to be on the bed before admission. Even if it isn't, having asked beforehand will help in getting it.

Possible Obstacles

Here are some things that others have said stood in their way of coordinating care

1. "I expect the doctor to coordinate care."

   Response: <u>The doctor may not know about what helped at home or at another treatment setting. You have to tell him or her</u>. You should give the doctor a list of medicines, how they are taken (such as pills, suppositories or injections, and so on), and times they are taken, and a list of what helps the patient swallow medicine. Doctors also don't know the specific elimination plan, mouth care routines, diets, or equipment that helped the person with cancer at home. <u>If you ask them to write this information as medical orders, then the nurses will do what the orders say</u>.

2. "I don't want the staff to think that I'm bossing them around."

   Response: <u>Nurses and doctors will welcome your information. These facts are important to the person's comfort and health</u>. Having written lists helps the nurses and doctors when they write this information in the medical record and order diet, equipment, and medicines.

3. "They don't have enough staff to do all the things I am asking for."

   Response: <u>Too few staff members is not an excuse. You have a right to expect good care</u>. If your requests are important for the care and comfort of the person with cancer, you may have to "make a fuss." You may also have to visit often to be sure things are happening as they should.

Think of *other* obstacles that could interfere with carrying out your plan

What additional road blocks could get in the way of doing the things recommended in this home care plan? For example, will the person with cancer cooperate? How will you explain what is needed to other people? Do you have the time and energy to carry out the plan?

You need to develop plans for getting around these road blocks. Use the four COPE ideas (creativity, optimism, planning, and expert information) in developing your plans. See the chapter on Solving Home Care Problems at the beginning of the book for a discussion of how to use the four COPE ideas in overcoming your obstacles.

Carrying Out and Adjusting Your Plan

How will you carry out your plan?

If possible, write your requests before the person you are caring for goes to a new treatment setting, and give them to the staff before or when he or she arrives. If the transfer happens too quickly for you to do this ahead of time, take your lists to the new medical staff as soon as possible after the transfer.

Checking on results

Check with the person you are caring for about whether the lists you made are being followed. Ask the nurses to see a copy of their orders, and check to be sure your lists are included.

If your plan doesn't work

If you are having difficulty giving your information to the right person, or if the staff is not using your information, ask a member of the health care team to help you. Involve them in solving the problem of coordinating care. Social workers are often good sources of help. They know the doctors and nurses and can give them your lists and ideas. You can also ask to talk with the charge nurse or head nurses about your concerns. If you still are unhappy about how care is being coordinated, ask to speak with the head nurse or patient advocate. Usually, such steps are not needed because the health care staff will want to continue using methods that worked at home to manage symptoms.

Coping with Anxiety

Overview of the
Home Care Plan for Coping with Anxiety

Understanding the Problem

What is anxiety?

Recognizing when a person is anxious

Anxiety related to cancer

What you can do to help

Family and friends can also become anxious

What you can hope to accomplish

When To Get Professional Help

Situations and symptoms that require professional help

What You Can Do To Help

Learn what thoughts are causing anxiety

Talk to someone who has been through the same situation

Increase pleasant, distracting activities

Increase companionship

Encourage use of relaxation techniques

Ask a physician for evaluation

Possible Obstacles

"My problems are real, so I have to worry about them."

"I can't stop anxious thoughts."

The family caregiver feels exhausted and doesn't have the energy to help other people with their emotional problems.

Carrying Out and Adjusting Your Plan

Work as a team

Plan in advance

Talk regularly about emotions

Don't expect change too fast

A Relaxation Technique

(Topics with an arrow in front of them are actions you can take or symptoms you can look for.)

Coping with Anxiety

[The information in this home care plan fits most situations, but yours may be different. If the doctor or nurse tells you to do something else, follow what they say.

The person with cancer is the one who will use the techniques in this home care plan. Your job is to help him or her make the best use of the techniques in this plan. The person with cancer should read this plan, and then the two of you should work together as a team. You can also use these techniques to control your own anxiety.]

Understanding the Problem

What is anxiety?

Anxiety is a common and normal response to new or stressful situations. Everyone has felt worried at various times in day-to-day life. For example, some people feel anxious or nervous before they interview for a new job, before talking to a group of people, or when they are worried about someone they love. Here are some different ways that people experience anxiety:

Nervousness

Tension

Panicky feelings

Fear

Feeling something bad is going to happen

Feeling like "I'm losing control"

When you are anxious you may also have physical symptoms like:

Sweaty palms

Upset stomach

Tight feelings in your stomach

Shaking or tremors

Difficulty breathing

Racing pulse

Hot and flushed in your face

Sometimes these feelings come and go fairly quickly. Other times these feelings last a long time.

Tension can help people to do something well. For example, many actors say that they have "butterflies in their stomach," or anxious moments, before they perform. Sometimes people actually enjoy the feelings of anxiety, like when they are watching a horse race or riding a roller coaster.

Anxiety

However, <u>when these feelings are very strong and contain fearful thoughts, they get in the way of everyday living. When they last a long time, they can prevent people from doing the things that are important to them. This is when people need to learn to manage anxiety better.</u>

Recognizing when a person is anxious

One of the difficult things about anxiety is that people may not know when they're experiencing it. They may think that they are just worried. But then, before they realize what is happening, they are experiencing serious anxiety symptoms.

<u>Sometimes the person with cancer doesn't realize how anxious he or she is becoming, but family and friends do. Family and friends can help by pointing out what is happening early, and they can help the person with cancer control the anxiety before it gets out of hand.</u>

Anxiety related to cancer

When people are told they have cancer, it often makes them feel anxious. Some feel afraid, nervous, and even overwhelmed. Others may feel panicky, as if they have lost control of their lives. These are normal reactions.

Many people with cancer experience anxiety during their illness. Anxiety can be caused by:

Worries about medical procedures

Fear of being a burden to family and friends

Pain and discomfort

Fear of getting sicker

A side effect of cancer treatment medicines

<u>Anxiety can make the symptoms of cancer more intense</u>. For example, a person who is in pain usually reports more severe pain when he or she is feeling anxious.

Although some anxiety is normal for people with cancer, it can become so severe that it interferes with their ability to cope with the illness. Anxiety may make some people reluctant to visit the doctor and may even make them think of dropping out of treatment. Severe anxiety can also seriously reduce the quality of life of the person with cancer.

What you can do to help

<u>Controlling anxiety is primarily in the hands of the person with cancer. You should work with him or her as a team to control and reduce the anxiety</u>.

You should not feel guilty or responsible if, in spite of your best efforts, the person with cancer is very anxious. If the anxiety is severe, a professional may be needed who can use special techniques such as anti-anxiety medicines or stress management techniques.

Family and friends can also become anxious

Family and friends caring for someone with cancer can also become anxious. Sometimes it is because they worry about the person's illness and their own ability to cope effectively with all the stress involved. Sometimes it is because the anxiety of the person with cancer makes them anxious. Poor communication between the person with cancer and family and friends can also be a source of anxiety for everyone. Therefore, you should read this home care plan both to help the person with cancer and also to help yourself.

What you can hope to accomplish

Since anxiety is a normal response to new or stressful situations, don't expect to totally eliminate all anxiety. What you and the person with cancer can do together is prevent anxiety from becoming so severe and so long lasting that it seriously degrades his or her quality of life or interferes with receiving needed cancer treatments.

Your goals are to:

accept that some anxiety is both normal and understandable,

help the person with cancer to get professional help for anxiety when that is necessary,

help the person with cancer learn about his or her anxiety and to manage it as much as possible, and

use this home care plan for yourself, if anxiety is interfering with your ability to help your loved one.

When To Get Professional Help

The first question you should ask is whether professional help is needed. You should urge the person with cancer to call the doctor, nurse, psychologist, or social worker for anxiety (or do so yourself) if he or she:

1. Is seriously considering dropping out of treatment, skipping treatments, or avoiding visits to the doctor because of anxiety.
2. Has a history of severe anxiety requiring professional help or therapy and is feeling very anxious now.
3. Has a much lower quality of life because of anxiety symptoms.

Anxiety

Professional help is needed if anxiety symptoms are interfering with daily activities or are very upsetting to the person with cancer.

Some people are hesitant to ask for help with emotional problems because they don't want to appear "crazy." They should understand that <u>being upset during a major illness is normal, and so is getting help for these problems</u>.

It is best to start with the physician treating the cancer or a family physician who knows the person with cancer and the treatments he or she is receiving. Ask for an evaluation of possible causes of the anxiety and recommendations for treatment or referral.

Physicians can evaluate whether a change in the cancer treatment or medicines is needed or whether to prescribe anti-anxiety medicines. Physicians can also make referrals to mental health professionals such as psychologists, psychiatrists, social workers, and nurse counselors.

<u>If you are not sure whether professional help is needed, ask a nurse or social worker for guidance.</u>

(<u>Also, be alert to whether family members need help because of anxiety. If their anxiety is severe, they may need help just as the person with cancer does</u>.)

Call the doctor, nurse, or social worker if any of the following symptoms persist for several days

Severe problems falling or staying asleep several days in a row

Feelings of dread and serious apprehension for several days

Trembling, twitching, and feeling "shaky"

Fluttering stomach with nausea and diarrhea

Increased heart rate or feeling a rapid pulse

Wide mood swings that you cannot control

Shortness of breath

Some of these symptoms could be caused by cancer or side effects of the treatments as well as by anxiety. The physician treating the person with cancer can evaluate what is causing these symptoms.

What You Can Do To Help

If it's not an emergency, here are six things you can do working as a team with the person with cancer. Always start with the first one— being sure about what thoughts are causing the anxiety:

find out what thoughts are causing the anxiety,

encourage talking to someone who has been through the situation causing the anxiety, increase pleasant, distracting activities,

increase companionship,

encourage use of relaxation techniques, and

ask a physician for an evaluation.

➤ **Try to find out exactly what thoughts are making him or her anxious.** Understanding the thoughts that are causing the anxiety is the key to controlling it.

Anxiety has two parts: thoughts and feelings. Worried thoughts lead to nervous feelings. Nervous feelings can lead to more worried thoughts and so on. To stop this cycle, you first need to find out what thoughts are causing the anxiety and why those thoughts are making him or her nervous.

For example, he or she may say going into the hospital is upsetting, but, when you ask what it is about the hospital that makes it upsetting, you may learn that he or she is afraid of being left alone. On the other hand, another person may be concerned about paying the bills. Sometimes you won't be able to find an exact reason; this is when professional help may be useful.

If the person is anxious about medical procedures, try to find out exactly what it is about the procedure that is upsetting. Is it needles, pain, being alone, being naked, being in an enclosed space? If the person cannot explain it, ask: "How would you change the procedures so that they don't make you so upset?"

If the person is anxious about receiving medical information, try to find out exactly what kind of news would likely cause the person to be upset. Is it being told to have more treatments? Having to go into the hospital? The prospect of being unable to do certain things in the future?

It is important to be tactful and sensitive when asking these types of questions. Just talking about the upsetting event may make the person even more upset.

➤ **Getting the facts can help a person feel less anxious.** For example, if he or she is worried about whether the doctor will say that the disease has progressed, you may learn that the doctor will not know whether the cancer is responding to treatment for another 8 weeks. Or, if he or she is upset by needles, you may learn that the test the doctor has ordered does not use needles.

➤ **When you get the facts, you may also discover that there are ways to "get around" a problem that is making the person anxious.** For example, if the anxiety is about needle sticks in the veins, blood could be drawn with a small prick on the finger. Or, if he or she is worried about being alone during chemotherapy or a test, you can plan to be with them during that time.

Anxiety

➤ **Encourage the person with cancer to talk to someone who has been through a similar situation.** It is often reassuring to hear about what happened to someone else and how that person reacted during a stressful experience. It helps the person with cancer to know that he or she is not alone and that someone else got through it. This can make the future seem more manageable, even if the experience was difficult for the other person.

When you talk to someone who has been through a similar situation be sure to involve the person with cancer. There is a possibility that these discussions will make him or her more upset. Therefore, it is important that he or she agree to and help plan the meeting or telephone call. You should choose the person you talk to carefully since some people can be more reassuring than others. In general, though, most people find that talking to someone who has been through the same experience reduces worry and anxiety.

Most people who have made it through scary experiences are happy to talk to others about their experiences. The treatment team may be able to refer you to a person or to a support group where you can find a person who has had similar experiences.

➤ **Increase pleasant, distracting activities.** Helping the person with cancer to think about and do things that are pleasant and relaxing can help reduce anxiety.

The home care plan for Maintaining Positive Experiences guides you in planning and carrying out three types of enjoyable activities: activities with other people, activities that give a sense of accomplishment, and activities that are especially involving so as to displace thoughts about the situation that is making him or her anxious.

➤ **Increase companionship and time spent with friends and family who care.** Being with family and friends that the person with cancer knows and enjoys is an excellent way to take attention away from what is causing the anxiety. It can also give family and friends the opportunity to express caring and love for him or her.

The home care plan for Getting Companionship and Support from Family and Friends guides you in developing plans to increase the amount of support and help the person with cancer receives from other people. Knowing that other people care and are available to help when needed gives people strength and confidence in facing frightening experiences.

➤ **Encourage the person with cancer to use relaxation techniques.** <u>Relaxation is a skill which can be used to counteract anxiety</u>. You can't be anxious and relaxed at the same time. When you do things that make the person with cancer feel relaxed, anxiety decreases.

<u>There are many ways to feel more relaxed. The person with cancer should choose a way that is comfortable</u>. Prayer or meditation helps many people when they are in tense situations. Many people are relaxed by certain kinds of music. Walking or mild exercise can reduce anxiety, too.

There are also special relaxation exercises and tapes which are available commercially. These programs teach relaxation as a skill. With practice, people can learn to relax their muscles more than they usually would. They can then learn to use this skill when they are in tense situations. Oncology nurses, doctors, psychologists, and social workers are often familiar with relaxation techniques and may be able to recommend a program, book, or audio-cassette tape.

The last section of this home care plan explains how to use and practice relaxation techniques. It is important that people practice these skills because the better the person with cancer is at becoming relaxed, the better he or she will be able to control anxiety.

➤ **Ask a physician for an evaluation and treatment recommendations.** <u>If anxiety does not improve in spite of your efforts to help, then you can encourage the person with cancer to discuss the problem with a physician</u>. Contact the physician treating the cancer or a family physician who knows about the medical situation and treatments.

Physicians can help in three ways:

1. They can assess whether the side effects of the disease or treatments may be causing the anxiety. They can then consider changes in the treatment, if it's appropriate.

2. They can assess whether anti-anxiety medicines should be prescribed. People with cancer should only take anti-anxiety medicine after consulting with a physician who is familiar with their cancer diagnosis and treatments. These medicines may cause problems when combined with other medicines.

3. They can assess whether referral to a mental health professional is needed. If so, they can help with a referral.

Anxiety

Possible Obstacles

Here are some obstacles that other people like you have faced in helping a person with cancer deal with anxiety

1. "My problems are real. I have to face them even if they make me anxious."

   Response: Agree that the problems are real. <u>A certain amount of anxiety about them is normal and understandable</u>. However, research and experience shows that <u>severe anxiety interferes with the ability to solve problems</u>. Managing anxiety makes problem solving easier. This home care plan will help to prevent anxiety from becoming severe.

2. "I can't stop the thoughts that make me anxious. They keep coming back and racing around my head."

   Response: It's scary to feel like you can't control your thoughts. However, there are some techniques to try which may reduce or even stop them. <u>In the home care plan for Coping with Depression, there is a section on stopping negative thoughts. These can work for anxiety, too</u>.

3. You (the family caregiver) are feeling exhausted and frustrated, so it is difficult for you to help other people with their emotional problems.

   Response: <u>Spending a lot of time with someone who is very anxious can be stressful and can even make you anxious, too</u>. You need to take time for yourself—to deal with your own problems. Use the home care plans for Maintaining Positive Experiences, Getting Companionship and Support from Family and Friends, Coping with Depression, and Coping with Anxiety for yourself as well as for the person you are caring for. You should also involve as many people as possible in carrying out this home care plan. More support will help both of you.

Think of _other_ obstacles that could interfere with carrying out your plan

What additional road blocks could get in the way of doing the things recommended in this home care plan? For example, will the person with cancer cooperate? Will other people help? How will you explain your needs to other people? Do you have the time and energy to carry out the plan?

You need to develop plans for getting around these road blocks. Use the four COPE ideas (creativity, optimism, planning, and expert information) in developing your plans. See the chapter on Solving Home Care Problems at the beginning of the book for a discussion of how to use the four COPE ideas in overcoming your obstacles.

Carrying Out and Adjusting Your Plan

Carrying out your plan

Your first step is to talk this plan over with the person with cancer. You are a team. You should agree on what you will do together to try to manage anxiety.

If you think that anxiety is likely at certain times, make plans for what to do at these times to prevent anxiety from building up. It is always easier to help someone manage anxiety before it is serious and before he or she feels overwhelmed by it.

Stay alert to the possibility that professional help may be needed. Review regularly the questions in the When To Get Professional Help section of this plan. Seek help if the anxiety seriously interferes with the ability of the person with cancer to complete treatment or if it is seriously hurting his or her quality of life.

Checking on results

Talk regularly with the person with cancer about emotional feelings just as you do about physical feelings. Some people find it helpful to rate their anxiety on a 10-point scale, with zero being "no anxiety" and 10 being "the worst anxiety ever experienced." Keeping a daily log of anxiety levels takes a little extra effort, but by keeping track of it, you can deal with it before it gets serious, and it can save a lot of energy later.

If the plan doesn't work

Ask if you are expecting change too fast. It usually takes time to change someone's anxiety level. Look for small improvements at first. Remember: Your efforts may be successful even if they just stop the anxiety from getting worse.

If these techniques do not seem to be helping and the person with cancer has been feeling anxious for several weeks, then you should get professional help.

Anxiety

A Relaxation Technique

Many persons with cancer have found relaxation techniques helpful. These techniques can be used anytime—even for short periods of time. Try this exercise yourself to see how it feels and works for you. This will help you to support the person with cancer in using these techniques.

Relaxation should be practiced once a day, but not within an hour after a meal since digestion may interfere with the ability to relax certain muscles.

The person with cancer should read this exercise. He or she may want you to help. If so, you can read these instructions out loud.

1. Sit quietly in a comfortable position (such as in an easy chair or sofa) and practice this exercise when you are not feeling rushed.

2. Close your eyes.

3. Deeply relax your muscles, beginning with the face and going throughout the entire body (shoulders, chest, arms, hands, stomach, legs) and ending with the feet. Allow the tension to "flow out through your feet."

   Now concentrate your attention on your head, and relax your head even further by thinking, "I'm going to let all the tension flow out of my head. I'm letting go of the tension, and I'm letting warm feelings of relaxation smooth out the muscles in my head and face. I'm becoming more relaxed."

   Repeat these same steps for different parts of your body: your shoulders, arms, hands, chest, abdomen, legs, and feet. Do this slowly—spend enough time to feel more relaxed before going on to the next part of the body.

4. When the body feels very relaxed, concentrate on your breathing. Become aware of how rhythmic and deep your breathing has become. Breathe slowly and deeply. Breathe through your nose. As you breathe out, say the word "calm" silently to yourself. Slowly take a breath in. Now slowly let it out and silently say "calm" to yourself. Repeat this with every breath. It helps you to relax more if you concentrate on just this one word "calm." Continue breathing deeply, becoming more and more relaxed.

5. Continue this exercise for 10 to 15 minutes more. Remain relaxed and breathing slowly. At the end of the exercise, open your eyes slowly to become adjusted to the light in the room, and sit quietly for a few minutes.

   When it is over, ask yourself how relaxed you became and if there were any problems. One problem can be drifting and distracting thoughts. If this happens at the next session, think to yourself, "Let relaxation happen at its own pace." If a distracting thought occurs, let it pass. Let it fly away like a bird. Don't fight it. Concentrate more on the word "calm." Let the thought drift by and repeat "calm" over and over again as your breathing gets slower and deeper—as you relax more and more.

6. Do these exercises regularly—once a day is best. In the beginning, it may help to have someone else give you the instructions. You can record these instructions on an inexpensive tape recorder and play them when you are relaxing. If you prefer, you can record yourself giving the instructions and use that.

7. When practicing, choose a time when you will not be disturbed. Tell the other people in your household what you are doing and ask them to be quiet during the exercise.

8. After you become skilled at this exercise, you will find that it is easy to apply when you are getting tense. For example, if you are feeling tense while waiting to see the doctor or for a treatment, you can easily close your eyes for a few minutes and use this exercise to relax and feel calm.

9. It's a good idea to learn this relaxation technique early—before anxiety becomes severe. It can then help to keep severe anxiety from happening.

Coping with Depression

Overview of the
Home Care Plan for Coping with Depression

Understanding the Problem

Depression is common among persons with cancer

How a person acts when depressed

Causes of depression

What you can do as a caregiver

Family and friends can also become depressed

When To Get Professional Help

Symptoms that indicate that professional help is needed

How to get professional help

What You Can Do To Help

Taking care of your own emotional needs when living with a depressed person

How to react to a person who is depressed

How to prevent or decrease depression

Possible Obstacles

"I don't want your help."

"It's normal to be depressed in my situation."

"It's no use trying."

Carrying Out and Adjusting Your Plan

Work as a team

Use these techniques early

Plan in advance and persist

Talk regularly with him or her about feelings

Watch to see if professional help is needed

Don't expect change too fast

Techniques for Controlling Negative Thoughts

Thought stopping

Arranging a time and place for negative thinking

Distraction

Arguing against negative thoughts

Solving day-to-day problems that are causing stress

(Topics with an arrow in front of them are actions you can take or symptoms you can look for.)

Coping with Depression

[The information in this home care plan fits most situations, but yours may be different. If the doctor or nurse tells you to do something else, follow what they say.

The person with cancer is the one who will use the techniques in this home care plan. Your job is to help him or her make the best use of these techniques. The person with cancer should read this plan, and then the two of you should work together as a team. You can also use these techniques to control your own depression.]

Understanding the Problem

The stress of dealing with an illness like cancer can cause many uncomfortable feelings such as depression. Sometimes we are able to get over "the blues" after a short time. But sometimes these feelings last a long time and can severely hurt the quality of a person's life. When a person is sad, discouraged, pessimistic, or despairing for several weeks or months, and when these feelings interfere with being able to manage day-to-day affairs, we say that he or she is suffering from depression. Depression can last a long time if the person doesn't do something to stop it.

In addition to feelings of sadness, the symptoms sometimes include problems with appetite, sleeping, having the energy to do things, and problems paying attention to things. Alcohol abuse, especially if it is new or worse since the illness, may be a sign of depression. Sometimes a depressed person also thinks about suicide as a way out.

If the person with cancer is depressed, he or she will have problems coping with their illness and the impact it has on their life.

Depression works like a downward spiral. The person feels down, so he or she doesn't put energy into solving problems. When the problems get worse, they can cause the person to feel worse. And so on and so on. Somehow this has to be interrupted. Some kind of change has to happen, or the person will have these feelings for a long time.

Depression can be a side effect of some medicines, or it can be caused by chemical imbalances in the body due to the cancer. When this happens, changes in medical treatments may help the depression.

In this home care plan, we discuss some ways to tell when a depressed person must seek medical help. We also discuss some ways that you can help a depressed person limit or manage depression. Your help is valuable to a person feeling depressed, but it is also important that he or she practice certain self-help strategies. We discuss ways that you and the person with cancer can work together as a team to deal with depression.

Some depression is a normal response to the stresses and uncertainties of chronic illness. <u>Don't expect to get rid of all of these feelings. However, you can help to limit the length and severity of depression</u>.

As a caregiver, you can help prevent feelings of sadness or discouragement from becoming severe or continuing for long periods of time. <u>Working as a team will help both of you keep depressed feelings under control</u>. If the symptoms become severe, you can help the person with cancer get professional help.

(Living with a person who is depressed can be stressful and can even lead to your becoming depressed. <u>It is important to pay attention to your own emotional health if you are to do your best as a caregiver</u>.)

Your goals are to:

work as a team with the person with cancer to manage depressed feelings and thoughts,

keep an eye out for early depressive symptoms and help the person with cancer to manage depression early before the symptoms become severe, and

take care of your own emotional needs when living with a person who is depressed.

When To Get Professional Help

Symptoms that indicate that professional help is needed

<u>If any of the following is occurring, you should get assistance from a health professional</u>.

➤ **He or she is talking about hurting or killing him- or herself.** <u>Suicide is not common among persons with cancer, although anyone who talks about suicide should be taken seriously</u>. If you are not sure, ask if he or she is thinking about suicide. Your asking won't make it more likely. If you think there is a possibility of suicide, this is a problem that requires professional assessment and help. Although it may be uncomfortable for you, you should seek professional assistance as soon as possible.

➤ **He or she has been depressed before this illness and has had at least two of the following symptoms consistently during the past 2 weeks:**

1. Feeling sad most of the day

2. Loss of interest in almost all daily activities

3. Difficulty paying attention to what he or she is doing and trouble making choices.

A person with a history of serious depression before the illness is vulnerable to depression after a major life stress. A serious illness like cancer often triggers depression in these people. Professional help is usually required to help them.

➤ **You notice wide mood swings from periods of depression to periods of agitation and high energy.** Some people who have wide, uncontrollable swings in mood may have a "manic-depressive" illness. They cycle between being depressed with low energy and having a great deal of energy with feelings of agitation or feeling "high." The moods often don't seem connected to what is going on around the person. This requires professional help to determine if medication is necessary.

➤ **Nothing you do seems to help, even those strategies that have worked in the past.**

How to get professional help

Getting help for depression is just like getting help for physical problems. Asking for help doesn't mean you are saying the person is crazy. The problem could be caused by the stress related to cancer or to the treatment itself. Or it could be an understandable reaction to the serious issues a person with cancer must face.

Some people are hesitant to ask for professional help with their emotional problems because they are embarrassed. They may think that seeing a psychologist, psychiatrist, or social worker means that they are weak or strange. Being upset during a major illness is normal. So is getting help for these problems. Professionals such as social workers, nurse counselors, clergy, psychologists, and psychiatrists are skilled and experienced in helping people deal with emotionally stressful experiences. They are there to help you with this kind of problem just like your family doctor is there to help with physical problems.

➤ **Ask for help from the physician who is treating the cancer, a family doctor, or another physician who is familiar with the medical treatments being given.** Physicians familiar with the person's medical condition and treatments can evaluate whether the depression is due to the disease or the treatment. If it's due to the treatment, then a change in treatment may be needed. Physicians can also evaluate whether anti-depression medications may help and can prescribe them if necessary.

> **Ask a mental health professional such as a social worker, psychologist, or psychiatrist for help.** Mental health professionals are experienced in helping people with many types of emotional problems. They can be especially helpful when there is a history of depression before the illness and when the depression is not due to the person's disease or treatments. Many psychologists, social workers, and other mental health professionals have experience working with people with cancer. They can be very helpful when depression is a reaction to the stress of the illness.

Changing depressed feelings takes time. It usually takes at least several sessions with a counselor or therapist before a person begins to feel better. It also takes time for medicines to work, and the doctor may need to adjust the doses before the medicines are helpful.

What You Can Do To Help

Take care of your own emotional needs when living with a depressed person

Many people are aware that depression happens frequently among persons with cancer. But fewer people recognize that family members and friends who care for someone with cancer also often experience depression during the illness. All the stress can make a person feel "burned out." When someone feels this frustrated, he or she won't be much help to another person.

Caregiving can be stressful. To do your best in this difficult role, you need to find ways to stay emotionally well yourself. Here are some things that you can do for your own emotional health:

> **Understand that it is not your fault if the person becomes depressed.** You should realize that you are not responsible if the person you are caring for becomes depressed. Depression can be caused by many things, including biological changes as well as changes in his or her life. Sometimes, especially if the depression is severe, only professionals can help. You should not feel guilty if, in spite of your best efforts, the person with cancer becomes or stays depressed.

> **Schedule positive experiences for yourself.** Keep doing things that make you feel good. Don't become so involved in your caring responsibilities that you neglect your own emotional health. Don't feel guilty about taking care of yourself. If you become overwhelmed, you won't be able to provide care and support. You will be a better caregiver if you take time to do things that you enjoy outside of your caring responsibilities. If you start feeling over-

whelmed, take time off to do the things you enjoy. Do this early. This can help prevent your becoming seriously depressed and give you the strength to carry on.

➤ **Get the companionship you need.** Remember that you need companionship. <u>Being with others is as important for you as for the person you are caring for</u>. Continue to do things with people you like and enjoy. This helps to prevent and manage your own "blues." If you feel yourself becoming depressed, seek out other people to talk to and do things with. Some people find it helpful to talk to other people about their problems. Others find it more helpful to talk about things that have nothing to do with their problems. This depends on how you feel and on the person you are talking to.

<u>You can get professional help for yourself, too</u>, if necessary.

How to react to a person who is depressed

➤ **Acknowledge that the person is depressed.** <u>One thing you should *not* do is to ignore the person's depression</u>. Sometimes people act as if the depression weren't there, either because they don't want to encourage it or because they don't want to deal with it. *This is wrong!* It is uncomfortable to acknowledge that someone you care for is depressed, but ignoring depression only makes it worse. The depressed person may feel that you do not care.

<u>You can be of most help early—before depression becomes severe</u>. If you ignore the early signs of depression, it is more likely to get out of hand, to seriously affect the quality of life of the person with cancer, and to require professional help.

➤ **Agree with correct and positive thinking.** Help correct those thoughts that seem wrong to you (see Techniques for Controlling Negative Thoughts at the end of this home care plan).

Of course, some of the depressed person's thoughts are correct. <u>You should make clear that you accept and agree with the correct parts. You are only disagreeing with the parts that seem wrong</u>. You can point out, in a supportive way, the incorrect thoughts.

A depressed person might say, "Nothing is going right." But there is usually something that is going okay. You can say, "I understand you're feeling discouraged, but let's think of some of the things that are going right."

The depressed person might say, "I'm a total failure." But you know that his or her whole life is not a failure. You might then say, "Maybe you've failed at some things, but think of all the things you have accomplished"—and then talk about several of them.

Depression

➤ **Encourage him or her to discuss the depression with a physician who understands the treatments being received or with a mental health professional.** See the discussion on asking for help from the physician who is treating the cancer in the section How To Get Professional Help in this home care plan.

How to prevent or decrease depression

Much of the work here has to come from the person with cancer. In this section, we describe a variety of methods that he or she can use to prevent or decrease depression. Both you and the person with cancer should read them carefully. If he or she cannot or does not want to read this plan, then explain the ideas and how you can help. These techniques work for most people. Your primary role is to be a team member by helping your loved one learn these strategies and then by being supportive and encouraging their use.

➤ **Help increase the number of pleasant, involving experiences for the person with cancer.** The home care plan for Maintaining Positive Experiences guides you in planning and carrying out three types of enjoyable activities: activities with other people, activities that give a sense of accomplishment, and activities that make the person feel good. Use that home care plan as part of your efforts to help the person with cancer combat depression.

➤ **Help increase the number of activities that the person with cancer does with other people.** Being with people you know and enjoy is an excellent way to take attention away from negative thoughts and feelings. It provides opportunities to think about one's own life in comparison to others and to recognize the good things in one's life. It provides opportunities to give as well as to receive help, to share experiences and perspectives, and to get help in dealing with problems that are making the person with cancer depressed. Most important is that other people can express caring and love for the person with cancer. Knowing that other people care and are available to help when needed gives people strength and confidence when facing an uncertain future.

Three types of people can be especially helpful for persons with cancer. Make a list of friends and family members using the following categories. Then use the home care plan for Getting Companionship and Support from Family and Friends to think of ways to be with these people.

1. People who are sympathetic and understanding

2. People who give good advice and who can help solve problems

3. People who can turn his or her attention away from problems and toward pleasant experiences.

The home care plan for Getting Companionship and Support guides you in developing plans to increase support and help from other people.

➤ **Encourage him or her to set reasonable, attainable goals.** Depressed people tend to set goals that are too high, and when they don't reach their goals, they tend to become even more depressed. When you plan positive experiences, be sure that your goals are reasonable. It is better to set a low goal and accomplish more than you expected than to set too high a goal and fail.

➤ **Support his or her efforts to control repetitive, negative thoughts and to substitute positive experiences and thoughts.** When the person with cancer tells you that he or she needs to do something to "break out" of depressive thoughts, you can help by encouraging and becoming involved in the activities. This can be as simple as talking about something pleasant or doing an activity together.

Five techniques for controlling negative thoughts are explained at the end of this home care plan. They are:

1. Thought stopping—to control repetitive negative thinking

2. Arranging a plan and time for negative thinking—to control and limit negative thoughts

3. Distraction—to take attention away from negative thoughts

4. Arguing against negative thinking—to show yourself how unreasonable your negative thoughts are

5. Solving day-to-day stressful problems that can be a cause of negative thoughts.

➤ **Make a plan to let the person with cancer know when you think he or she is doing things which may lead to depression.** This helps him or her to manage the depression early, before it becomes severe. Some people find it easiest to use a code word or phrase that the two of you agree on to point out depressed thinking. However you do it, a gentle reminder for him or her to stop and think about negative thoughts and unrealistic goal setting can help give a way to prevent the depression from setting in.

Possible Obstacles

Think about obstacles that could stop you from carrying out your plan and about how you will deal with them.

Here are some obstacles that other people, like yourself, have faced in helping a person with cancer deal with depression

1. "I don't want your help. Leave me alone."

   Response: Explain that you can't do anything without cooperation. He or she must participate in the home care plan if it is going to be effective. <u>Explain that you will not do anything without his or her agreement and cooperation</u>. Next, have him or her read this home care plan. Discuss it together and agree on what you will try first. Start small—with something that is easy to do—and then evaluate the results. If the depression is so severe that the person with cancer doesn't even want to try, professional help may be needed.

2. "My problems are real! It's normal to be depressed in my situation."

   Response: Agree that the problems are real and some depression is normal. But suggest that getting stuck in the feeling of depression can interfere with dealing with the problems that are causing the depression. Explain that the goal is to keep a balance between positive and negative thoughts. <u>The problems are real, but many of the good things in life are also real and should get equal attention</u>.

3. "Nothing will help, so it's no use trying."

   Response: Urge him or her to give it a try! There is nothing to lose and a good deal to gain. <u>Start with things that are easiest to do. Then judge if these ideas are helpful</u>. If the person with cancer is so depressed that he or she can't even try, then professional help is probably needed.

Think of *other* obstacles that could interfere with carrying out your plan

What additional road blocks could get in the way of doing the things recommended in this home care plan? For example, will the person with cancer cooperate? Will other people help? Do you have the time and energy to carry out the plan?

You need to develop plans for getting around these road blocks. Use the four COPE ideas (creativity, optimism, planning, and expert information) in developing your plans. See the chapter on Solving Home Care Problems at the beginning of the book for a discussion of how to use the four COPE ideas in overcoming your obstacles.

Carrying Out and Adjusting Your Plan

Carrying out your plan

➤ **Talk this plan over with the person with cancer.** <u>Together you should agree on what you can do together to manage depression</u>. It is important to work as a team when dealing with these problems. Sometimes the support and the feeling of being on a team is in itself helpful to a depressed person.

➤ **Use these techniques early.** <u>Look for beginning signs of depression and put your plan into action then</u>—don't wait until depression is severe. The techniques discussed in this plan have helped severely depressed persons, but usually as part of professional treatment. As a caregiver, you can help most before depression becomes severe.

➤ **Plan in advance what you will do to manage depression.** If you know that the person with cancer is likely to be depressed at certain times based on past experience, then make plans for what you will do to prevent depression from building up.

➤ **Persist.** Even if the person with cancer continues to feel depressed, don't give up. You are probably preventing the depression from getting worse. <u>Keep working cooperatively with the depressed person</u>. If you are working together, these ideas can only help.

Checking on results

➤ **Talk regularly with the person with cancer about his or her feelings.** Although it may be difficult for you at first, let the person with cancer know that you understand that depression can happen during this illness. If you show that you are comfortable talking about feelings, the person with cancer is more likely to let you know early on if he or she is experiencing depressive symptoms.

It may seem scary at first to talk to a depressed person about what is upsetting him or her. But it's important to do this because it shows that you care, and it helps you to work together, as a team, to control the depressed thoughts and feelings.

➤ **Watch for indications that professional help is needed.**

If the plan doesn't work

Ask if you are expecting change too fast. It usually takes time to manage depression. Look for a small improvement at first. Remember: Your efforts may be successful even if they just keep the depression from getting worse.

If these techniques do not seem to be helping and the person with cancer has been feeling very depressed for several weeks, review this home care plan to be sure you have tried all of the ideas. If so, you should encourage the person with cancer to seek professional help.

Techniques for Controlling Negative Thoughts

Thought stopping

One of the hard things about depression is that it's so easy to get stuck in a whirlwind of negative thinking. Suddenly you may find depressing thoughts going around and around in your head. It doesn't take long for this to make you feel bad; and then it may seem like you can't stop it. But you *can!*

The thought-stopping technique helps you to "snap out of it" when that whirlwind of negative thoughts first starts. If you catch it early, you can keep it from getting you too upset. The trick is to do this when you *first* notice a negative thought.

When you first feel yourself in the negative-thinking whirlwind, try one of these techniques:

➤ **Yell "STOP" really loudly in your mind.** Yell STOP when you scream STOP in your mind; pretend it is very loud. The idea is to wake you up, to make you aware that you're in danger of getting stuck in negative thoughts. You might start this by going to a place by yourself and shouting STOP out loud. Practice it this way until you can do it in your mind alone.

➤ **Visualize a big red STOP sign.** Try to see it clearly, and then get your mind on something else. Think of what a STOP sign looks like. Make sure you see it as a red sign. Practice seeing it in your mind so that you can bring it to mind easily. Now whenever you catch yourself starting negative thoughts, think of this image and stop yourself.

➤ **Slap yourself on the wrist with a rubber band.** Another way to remind yourself to stop is to gently slap your wrist with a rubber band. This isn't to punish yourself. It's to give you a physical reminder to stop the thoughts.

➤ **Splash some water on your face.** Splashing water in your face is another way to wake yourself up from the negative thinking. Pay attention to how the water makes you feel. And stop your negative thoughts.

➤ **Get up and move to a new spot.** Getting up and moving to a new spot gives you a change of scenery. You can use the new surroundings to help you think about other things.

You have to fight the negative thoughts. Maybe several of these techniques together will work for you.

When you're depressed, you may look at techniques for stopping these thoughts and say, "That's silly. It could never work." Actually, research has shown that they *can work.* Give them a try!

Arranging a time and a place for negative thinking

This technique allows you to think about negative things, but puts *you* in control of when and where you do this thinking.

➤ **Find a negative-thinking "office."** This can be a room, a chair, or just a certain window. Make this the only place you let yourself think about all of the negative things.

Your "office" space can be any place you choose. Don't, however, make it your bed or your seat where you eat. These need to be "safe zones." Now you should try to only think your negative thoughts in this one place.

➤ **Schedule a time each day when you plan to think your negative thoughts.** Scheduling a time to think about your negative thoughts helps you to take control of them. You might not be able to control all negative thinking, especially in the beginning. But this technique will gradually help you to get control over your negative thinking.

Don't make this time around mealtimes, just before you go to sleep, or just before you expect to see people. These should be relaxing times. Make this time no more that 15 minutes. At the end of 15 minutes, stop. You can continue tomorrow.

Distraction

You can't think two things at once. When you start thinking negative thoughts, get your mind involved in another activity which "pushes out" or replaces the negative thinking. Try one of these ideas:

➤ **Take a vacation in your mind.** Close your eyes and think about your favorite spot. Spend a couple minutes there on a mental vacation. Relax and enjoy it.

➤ **Mental time travel into the future.** Think of something that you are looking forward to. Imagine that it is happening. Think of how nice it is to be there.

> When you take your mental vacation or time travel to something you're looking forward to, really try to work your imagination. Think about as many details as possible.

> What does it feel like? Is it a warm breeze? Imagine how it feels on your skin.

> What does it sound like? Are there waves gently crashing on the beach? Are people laughing, or is music playing? Imagine it as clearly and vividly as you can.

> What does it look like? Is the sky clear and blue? Or are you in a room? Imagine what the room looks like. Try to see it as completely as you can.

> What does it smell like? Is it the salty smell of the ocean? Maybe you smell the fragrances of a garden or a big dinner. Make it as clear as you can.

> What does it taste like? Are you drinking a nice cool drink? Feel it in your mouth. Taste it.

Use these exercises to fill your mind with as many pleasant details as you can. Think of as many as you can. This exercise is also helpful when you are feeling anxious and need help falling asleep.

➤ **Tension busting.** Use the relaxation exercises in the home care plan for Coping with Anxiety. Being relaxed helps you to think about pleasant things.

➤ **Do something you like.** Use the home care plan on Maintaining Positive Experiences. Really get yourself involved in an activity you like.

The idea of this exercise is to fill your mind up with positive thoughts and to have them crowd out the negative ones.

Arguing against negative thoughts

The idea of this exercise is to make yourself see both sides of the picture. Things aren't usually as bad as they first seem when you're depressed. But the only way to see the other side is to actively argue against it.

You can fight your negative thoughts. Challenge their accuracy. Every situation has at least two sides to it. When you're depressed, you probably only see the bad side. If you weren't depressed, you would usually think of both sides. This exercise forces you to actively take the other side. It is like having a debate with yourself.

➤ **Is your negative thought really true?** Make yourself be clear about what evidence supports it.

➤ **Now take the other side. Argue the exact opposite.** Think of every reason why your thought may not be true or may be exaggerated. Don't give up too easily. Really argue as if you were arguing with someone else.

When you're arguing with your negative thoughts, try to be as complete as possible. You may want to write down the answers to the following questions.

What is the evidence against my negative thought?

Are there any "facts" in my thinking which are really just assumptions?

Is my argument an example of "black and white" thinking? Are there shades of gray that I'm ignoring?

Is the negative side taking things out of context? Am I looking at the whole picture or just one small part of it?

Am I trying to predict the future, when I really know that I can't?

Try to punch as many holes in your "negative sides" argument as you can. Don't accept any illogical thinking at all.

Solve day-to-day problems that are causing you stress

Use a problem-solving approach to solving some of the day-to-day problems that are contributing to your feelings of depression, such as finding enough time to do housework, problems with family members, and so on.

The home care plan on Solving Home Care Problems at the beginning of this book explains how to use four problem-solving steps to deal with problems that are not included in this workbook. The four steps are:

➤ **Get information from cancer care experts about the problem and what you can do** (the kind of information that is in the home care plans)

➤ **Develop your plan in an orderly way,** including reviewing the facts, setting reasonable goals, and choosing the strategies that are the best balance between risk and benefit. When you encounter obstacles, you should:

➤ **Keep a positive outlook**, and

➤ **Be creative** by seeing the problem from someone else's perspective, asking other people for ideas, and rethinking your expectations.

You can remember these ideas with the word COPE:

C for being Creative

O for being Optimistic

P for Planning and

E for using Expert information.

Index

W

Waking up, 36, 98
Walking, 45, 212–213
  problems, 96
Watery eyes, 27
Weight gain, 94
Weight loss, 43, 44, 94
White blood cells, 30
Wigs, 147–148
Women
  communicating styles, 14
  sexual problems, 155, 158–160
World Health Organization, 94–95

Y

Yellow skin, 134